Diagnostic Imaging of Dogs and Cats

John P. Graham, MVB, MSc, DVR, MRCVS
Diplomate, ECVDI, Diplomate, ACVR

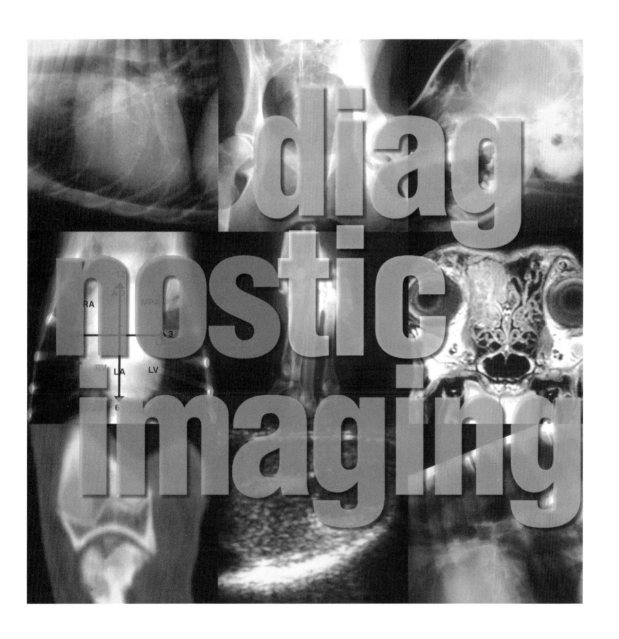

Nestlé PURINA Clinical Handbook Series

Published by The Gloyd Group, Inc.

Wilmington, Delaware

© 2002 by Nestlé Purina PetCare Company.

All rights reserved.

Printed in the United States of America.

Nestlé Purina PetCare Company: Checkerboard Square, Saint Louis, Missouri, 63188

First printing, 2002.

ISBN 0-9678005-7-9

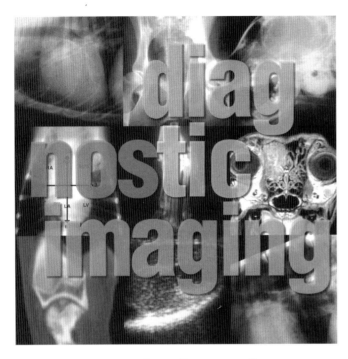

Diagnostic Imaging of Dogs and Cats

John P. Graham, MVB, MSc, DVR, MRCVS
Diplomate, ECVDI, Diplomate, ACVR

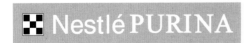

Nestlé PURINA

Clinical Handbook Series

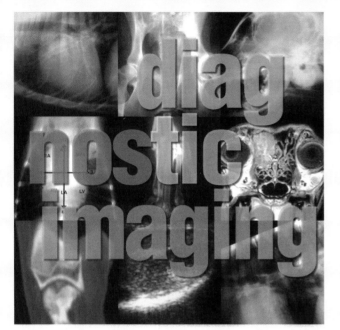

Wilhelm Conrad Roentgen discovered x-rays just over 100 years ago, and the first published radiograph was an image of his wife's hand. Within a few years radiographs were being used in veterinary medicine. Diagnostic radiology is now an integral part of veterinary practice. Imaging modalities such as ultrasound, computed tomography, magnetic resonance imaging, and nuclear medicine have expanded veterinary diagnostic capabilities and understanding of disease beyond Roentgen's wildest imaginings. A proliferation of new technologies has transformed the field of veterinary radiology into the broader field of veterinary diagnostic imaging.

The science (and art) of interpreting diagnostic images is the cornerstone of many diagnoses. Imaging tests have the advantage of being quick and noninvasive or minimally invasive. These technologies offer the ability to see inside the body and detect pathologic changes as well as evaluate organ function, which could otherwise be discovered only by surgery or necropsy. Imaging data complement and enhance the information obtained by clinical examination and other clinical tests.

In veterinary medicine, the two most important imaging modalities are radiography and ultrasound. Used alone or in combination, they allow the examination of almost any organ or body part. In addition, computed tomography, magnetic resonance imaging, and nuclear medicine are now available at most veterinary schools and are increasingly common in referral practices.

This handbook provides an overview of diagnostic imaging — predominantly radiology and ultrasonography — as it pertains to general small animal practice. Important principles and key abnormalities are outlined for each body part.

Part I addresses the process of image interpretation. **Part II** describes the imaging of the musculoskeletal system. **Part III** explores the unique demands of imaging the thorax and the abdomen and includes a chapter on abdominal ultrasound. **Part IV** displays the imaging challenges of specific canine and feline cases along with their diagnostic outcomes. The final section, **Part V**, contains a concise **Index of Figures** for easy reference to visual support; an imaging-specific **Glossary of Terms;** a list of **Suggested Reading** resources for more in-depth study; and a helpful **Subject Index** for quick access to particular conditions, techniques, and cases.

Part I

Interpreting diagnostic images produced by any modality requires a combination of skill and experience. The skill component can be developed by training and study, but experience can only be obtained over time. Regardless of the diagnostic imaging modality, a consistent systematic approach to interpretation is essential to accurate analysis and reliable diagnoses.

Radiologic interpretation is based on detecting alterations from normal. Changes in size, shape, margin, position, number, symmetry, and opacity are evaluated (*Figure 1*). The same process can be applied to other imaging modalities by substituting

- *opacity* for echogenicity in diagnostic ultrasound,
- *attenuation* in computed tomography,
- *signal intensity* in magnetic resonance imaging, and
- *radiopharmaceutical uptake* in nuclear medicine.

Thorough analysis of the images presented is essential to reaching an accurate diagnosis. The most reliable approach is to use a combination of two techniques. The observer should evaluate all of the body parts or components in the image sequentially. It is important to develop a checklist and always follow the list. This approach is especially useful for complex images, such as thoracic radiographs and abdominal ultrasound. Second, one should consider what diseases may affect a particular body part and evaluate the image for evidence of lesions. This is most useful when evaluating the musculoskeletal system, where structures are less complex. One must be careful, however, not to develop tunnel vision or search for what one thinks is the most likely diagnosis.

The process of lesion detection can be divided into three phases: **fixation, recognition,** and **diagnosis.** As the eye scans an image, a vast amount of information is presented to the brain. **Fixation** occurs when the eye focuses on a

Figure 1 Lateral radiograph of the abdomen of a cat. The five basic radiopacities are indicated: (1) *gas*, air outside the cat; (2) *fat*, the falciform ligament; (3) *soft tissue/fluid*, the liver; (4) *mineral*, bone of the lumbar spine; (5) *metal*, metallic clips used for a splenectomy.

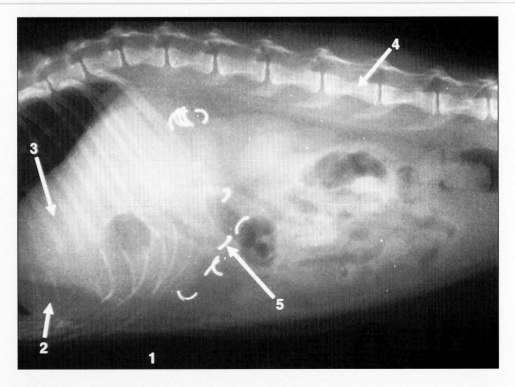

portion of the image. Factors that influence how the brain perceives this data include lighting conditions, image sharpness, and image contrast. Many optical illusions are based on the tendency of the brain to distort data presented to it by the eyes. In other words, what the eye sees is not always what the brain sees; and this disparity occurs frequently when viewing radiographs.

After an image has been presented to the brain, the second phase, lesion **recognition**, depends on a process of comparing the actual image with the expected normal appearance. This phase is affected by the experience of the observer; in effect, the quality and quantity of stored normal images in the brain. Other factors that may influence this phase include bias or prejudice on the part of the observer.

If the brain recognizes a lesion, then the third phase is **diagnosis**. In this phase the brain determines whether the lesion is real or not and what, if any, significance to ascribe to it. The interpretation phase may be affected by such factors as clinical suspicions or prejudices and observer experience.

This complex lesion detection process occurs very quickly. Many people spend a few minutes studying a radiograph, but in ultrasonography the brain is presented with 10 to 20 images *per second* to analyze. The intricacy of the process leaves it open to many sources of error. Poor viewing conditions, complacency, or inadequate attention may result in failure to fix the lesion. The brain may fail to recognize an abnormality as such, especially in inexperienced observers. A lesion may be dismissed as a normal anatomic variant or an artifact. Alternatively, an insignificant finding, an artifact, or normal variant may be interpreted as an important lesion.

The ability to quickly and confidently recognize normal structures distinguishes experienced radiologists from others when interpreting images. The observer's level of experience and any preconceived ideas about likely diagnoses have major impact on the detection process. Bias or preconceived ideas are also likely to result in an erroneous conclusion about the significance of a lesion. In all cases, regardless of experience, observers either under-read or over-read diagnostic images depending on their biases, per-

ceived consequences of a false-negative or false-positive diagnosis, and personality traits. Errors may also arise due to the phenomenon of "satisfaction of search," wherein, having discovered one or two lesions, the observer ceases the search for abnormalities and fails to detect additional lesions. This kind of error tends to compound itself because, if a lesion is not detected on the first examination, then it is likely to go undetected during later examinations as there is no impetus to look for it.

Interpretation of diagnostic images is an exacting process, and even highly skilled and experienced practitioners will make mistakes. A number of methods can be adopted to minimize errors. First, every effort should be made to achieve an optimum quality image. An accurate radiographic technique chart for all body parts should always be used. Processing artifacts can be minimized by good darkroom hygiene, careful attention to chemistry formulation, and routine maintenance and cleaning of processing tanks or the automatic processor. Radiographic variables, such as positioning and film or screen type, should be kept constant. If all studies performed are of diagnostic quality, then a strong foundation for interpretation has been established. For difficult cases, good-quality images are more likely to yield a diagnosis if submitted to a radiologist.

Again, the most important aspect of image interpretation is to use a systematic and exhaustive approach. The old adage, "More lesions are missed from not looking than from not knowing," is nowhere more true than in radiology. If possible, a quiet area with good quality view boxes should be set aside for radiographic interpretation; and distractions should be excluded. Similarly, a quiet room away from the bustle of the clinic should be used for performing ultrasound examinations. The effect of bias on interpretation in general practice, where the person evaluating the radiographs is also the attending clinician, is hard to avoid. It is important to be aware that the possibility of bias exists and attempt to exclude preconceived ideas about a particular case. When possible, seeking a second opinion from a colleague is valuable. Last, the observer should always ask, "What have I missed?" and review all findings before making a final decision.

Part II

The skeleton is in many ways ideally suited to radiographic examination. Bone readily absorbs x-radiation, resulting in images with very good contrast. The skeleton is limited, however, in range of responses to an insult, either producing more bone, removing bone, or a mixture of both. Therefore, when evaluating skeletal structures, careful attention to fine detail is essential. Many diseases appear similar radiographically; but subtle differences and features, such as lesion distribution, nonskeletal lesions, and signalment, are helpful in refining a diagnosis.

It is beneficial in musculoskeletal radiology to consider both generic changes and specific diseases. A useful analogy when exploring the radiographic diagnosis of skeletal disease is to think of osteoclasts and osteoblasts as demolition workers and builders and bone as the building site. Acute, active, and aggressive lesions—much like a building in the early stages of construction—appear quite untidy and disorganized. Chronic, inactive, and nonaggressive lesions appear well organized and orderly—like a finished building project.

Radiographic Quality

Radiographs can be obtained to evaluate the skeleton by different techniques, depending upon the personal preference of the reviewer. A technique using high kilovolt peak, kV(p), and low milliampere, mA, settings produces relatively gray images with limited inherent contrast, which can be tolerated as there is generally good contrast between bones and soft tissue. Bone structures appear well penetrated, and internal structures are clearly visible. A disadvantage is that soft tissues appear gray and dark. When using this kind of technique, it is essential to evaluate relatively dark areas of the image with a hot light.

Alternatively, a technique that uses a low kV(p) and high mA setting produces images with high contrast, the bones appearing relatively white. The kV(p) selected must produce an x-ray beam sufficiently powerful to penetrate bones, so that such detail as the inner margin of the cortex and medullary trabeculae can be appreciated. Soft tissues are generally easier to evaluate using this technique, and poorly mineralized new bone formation is also easier to see.

Either technique can be used depending on preference and the circumstances of the examination. Films of joints should be centered on the joint. Films of long bones should include the joints proximal and distal to the bone of interest. Care should be taken to achieve good positioning, and at least two orthogonal views must be obtained.

Benign or Nonaggressive Versus Aggressive or Malignant Lesions

Determining whether a skeletal lesion is aggressive or nonaggressive is a frequent diagnostic dilemma. Rather than simply a system with two or three classifications, the clinician should think of the classification of skeletal lesions as a continuous scale from nonaggressive to aggressive. Lesions may be characterized by bone destruction, new bone growth, or both. Each component should be evaluated to determine how long it has been present and how active it is.

Bone Destruction

Bone lysis, or destruction, is placed in one of three classifications based on the size of the holes in the bone. Large lesions (greater than 5 mm) are classed as *focal* or geographic (*Figure 2.1*). Lytic processes characterized by mid-sized holes (1 to 4 mm) are termed *moth-eaten*, and small

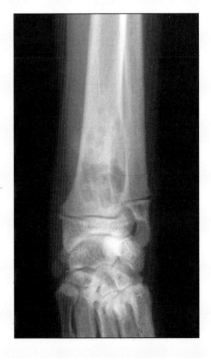

Figure 2.1 Craniocaudal view of the distal antebrachium of a 10-month-old jungle cat. There is a well-defined focal, or geographic, lytic lesion within the distal diaphysis and metaphysis of the radius. This was a bone cyst.

holes (less than 1 mm) are termed *permeative* (**Figure 2.2**). In general, the smaller and more numerous the holes, the more aggressive the lesion.

The observer should evaluate the margins of the holes. Well-defined, sharply demarcated borders suggest a nonaggressive lesion. Poorly defined and indistinct margins indicate an active, relatively aggressive lesion.

The zone of transition at the junction between the lytic lesion and normal bone should be evaluated. A sharp, well-defined transition suggests a nonaggressive process. If a sclerotic rim of bone is present at the junction of normal and abnormal bone, then that usually indicates a chronic process that the skeleton is attempting to contain. A broad zone of transition, for which it is difficult to say definitively where bone is normal or abnormal, is consistent with an aggressive process.

New Bone Formation

Bone production usually occurs on the periosteal surface of the cortex in response to lifting or tearing of the fibrous periosteum. Periosteal new bone should be evaluated for shape, margination, and definition (**Figures 2.3 to 2.6**). Lamellated new bone consists of multiple layers, appearing much like a cross section of an onion; it is usually chronic and the result of repeated insults. Lamellated bone may be seen at the edge of an expansile lesion where repeated growth spurts lift the periosteum from the original cortex, and then the new bone forms in layers. A palisade type of new bone formation has a ragged margin and resembles a picket fence in appearance. This appearance is associated with a lesion that is at least moderately aggressive. Solid homogeneous periosteal new bone indicates a chronic and probably inactive process. The so-called "sunburst" pattern of new bone formation is relatively uncommon and appears as radiating spicules of poorly defined new bone.

The degree of mineralization of new bone is a useful and reliable indicator of the age of a lesion and, to a lesser extent, of the degree of aggression. Poorly mineralized new bone is almost always recently formed. In adult animals, it takes approximately 10 days for mineralized new bone to become radiographically visible and, sometimes, only if using a hot light or by making an underexposed film. In juvenile animals, mineralization may happen more quickly; and new bone formation may be visible 5 to 7 days after an insult. Acute periosteal new bone may be so poorly mineralized that it is not visible without using a hot light. A relatively underexposed film may be helpful in detecting very

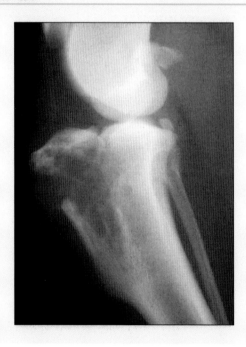

Figure 2.2 Lateral radiograph of the stifle of a rottweiler dog. Moth-eaten lysis of the tibial tuberosity is visible, as is a pathologic fracture of the weakened bone. Permeative lysis can be seen extending distally into the diaphysis of the tibia. This was an osteosarcoma.

poorly mineralized new bone. If the degree of mineralization of new bone is comparable to that of the original underlying cortical bone, then a chronic process is indicated.

The shape and definition of the margin of the new bone should also be evaluated. A useful rule of thumb is that, if it is impossible to trace the outline of the new bone with a sharp pencil, then it is classified as poorly defined and should be considered recent and active in nature. A well-defined edge indicates a chronic process, and a smooth margin indicates a chronic lesion that is completely remodeled and probably inactive. A well-defined irregular margin suggests a lesion that is chronic but probably active and likely to be mildly to moderately aggressive. Productive lesions often include both active and inactive areas of bone formation. In such cases, the lesion should be classified based on the most aggressive new bone.

The rate of change of a lesion is a useful indicator of the degree of aggression or malignancy. Serial radiographs obtained at 7- to 14-day intervals can be used to evaluate suspicious lesions, especially when the initial findings are equivocal. Aggressive lesions usually show a rapid rate of change, with clear evidence of progression of osteolysis and bone formation over a relatively short period of time.

Figure 2.3 Dorsoplantar view of the tarsus and metatarsus of a 3-year-old Dalmatian dog. The dog had suffered a degloving injury 6 weeks before presentation. There is mild soft tissue swelling. Palisade-type new bone formation is notable on the metatarsal bones. Irregularly marginated, palisade, well-defined new bone is also visible on the tarsal bones. This new bone appears chronic, active, and mildly aggressive. The lesion is consistent with periostitis due to soft tissue infection.

Figure 2.4 Craniocaudal view of the distal antebrachium of a 7-year-old Great Dane dog. New bone formation surrounds the distal diaphysis and metaphysis of the radius. The new bone is moderately well mineralized and slightly irregularly marginated. There is moth-eaten lysis within the distal radial metaphysis. This lesion is moderately aggressive. Diagnosis: osteosarcoma.

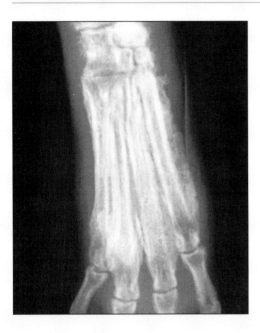

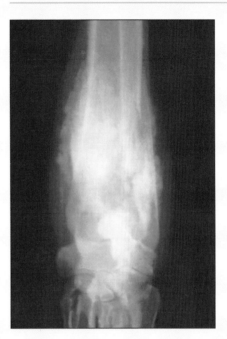

Figure 2.5 Craniocaudal view of the antebrachium of a 12-year-old domestic shorthair cat. Moderate soft tissue swelling surrounds the antebrachium. Irregularly marginated, ill-defined new bone, which is moderately to poorly mineralized, can be noted on the lateral aspect of the diaphysis of the ulna. Similar new bone formation is present on the proximal medial aspect of the radial diaphysis. This new bone formation is active and aggressive. Histologic diagnosis: squamous cell carcinoma.

Figure 2.6 Latero-medial view of the femur of a 4-month-old Labrador retriever puppy. Well-mineralized, smoothly marginated new bone surrounds the entire diaphysis of the femur. This new bone blends with the underlying femoral diaphysis. The new bone appears inactive and nonaggressive. Diagnosis: healed osteomyelitis.

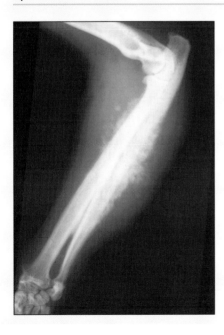

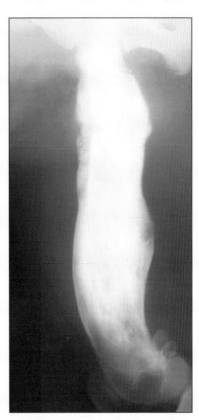

If serial radiographs demonstrate no change over a period of 4 to 6 weeks, then the lesion is almost certainly nonaggressive.

All of these changes are considered in deciding how aggressive a skeletal lesion is. Some lesions have both aggressive and nonaggressive features. A common example is an osteosarcoma, which may have moth-eaten and permeative lysis in the center of the tumor but well-organized, well-mineralized new bone at the periphery where the expanding tumor has lifted the periosteum. A lesion should be classified based on its most aggressive feature.

Neoplasia Versus Infection

Both neoplastic and infectious diseases affect the appendicular and axial skeleton, and the radiographic changes observed are often very similar or indistinguishable. Primary bone tumors in dogs are most commonly malignant and usually exhibit features indicating an aggressive nature. Fungal osteomyelitis may produce similar radiographic changes. Bacterial osteomyelitis has a variable appearance depending on the agent involved, age of the patient, and chronicity of the lesion.

Most primary malignant bone tumors in dogs are osteosarcomas (*Figures 2.7 to 2.9*), which more commonly

Figure 2.7 Mediolateral view of the proximal humerus of an 11-year-old mixed-breed dog. Moderately mineralized to well-mineralized new bone formation is notable at the caudal cortex of the proximal metaphysis of the humerus. There is increased opacity within the proximal humerus. This lesion is predominantly osteoproductive and is mildly aggressive. Histologic diagnosis: osteosarcoma.

Figure 2.8 Mediolateral view of the proximal femur of a 9-year-old German shepherd dog. A destructive lesion can be seen within the proximal metaphysis of the femur, which has well-defined margins. There are also multiple, small, focal, lytic lesions within the cortex. Well-mineralized, smoothly marginated, new bone formation is visible on the cranial cortex of the femur. This lesion appears moderately aggressive. Histologic diagnosis: osteosarcoma.

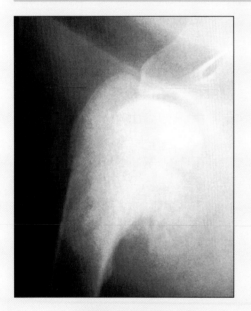

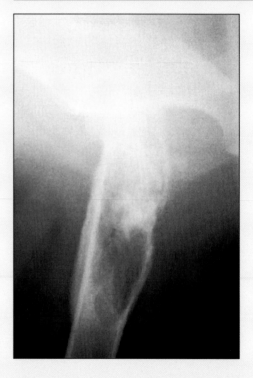

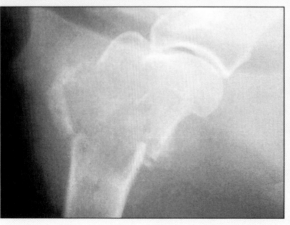

Figure 2.9 Mediolateral view of the proximal humerus of a 10-year-old golden retriever dog. There is an expansile destructive process with indistinct margins within the proximal metaphysis of the humerus. The lesion has weakened the bone, and pathologic fracture lines are present in the caudal and cranial cortices. There is also ill-defined, poorly mineralized, periosteal new bone on the caudal and cranial cortices. This lesion appears aggressive. Histologic diagnosis: osteosarcoma.

affect large and giant breed dogs. There is biphasic pattern of incidence, with peaks at approximately 1 year of age and at 7 years or older. The tumor has a predilection for the metaphyses of long bones, most commonly in the proximal humerus, distal radius, distal femur, and proximal and distal tibia. Typically, only a single bone is involved and the tumor does not cross joints or invade adjacent bones. The radiographic appearance varies from almost exclusively destructive to osteoproductive and all variants between. Appendicular lesions are most common, but the tumor also occurs in the axial skeleton. Pulmonary metastases are common but usually become radiographically visible only at late stages of the disease; skeletal metastases are uncommon. Other sarcomas, such as chondrosarcoma, fibrosarcoma, giant cell tumor, and hemangiosarcoma, also occur as primary bone tumors and are similar in appearance to osteosarcoma.

Metastatic skeletal neoplasia is relatively uncommon in companion animals. Lesions are more commonly seen with mammary tumors, prostatic carcinomas, and tumors originating in the lower urinary tract. The metastatic emboli are delivered to the bone by the blood supply, which determines the pattern of distribution. Metastasis may also occur by direct invasion from an adjacent soft tissue malignancy. This possibility should be considered if several adjacent bones are affected. In long bones, the lesions are typically diaphyseal rather than metaphyseal (*Figure 2.10*). The vertebral column and ribs are also common sites for metastatic neoplasia (*Figure 2.11*).

The distribution of bacterial osteomyelitis depends on the age of the animal and the origin of the infection. In skeletally immature animals, the long-bone blood supply differs because of the presence of the physes. The capillary sinuses on the metaphyseal side of the physis have sluggish blood flow due to the 180° turn that the blood makes. This is the site where hematogenously delivered bacterial emboli tend to settle. In immature animals, bacterial osteomyelitis most commonly occurs at the metaphysis or is associated with the epiphysis or joint.

Hematogenous osteomyelitis is uncommon in mature animals. The lesions are usually found in the diaphysis of long bones, just as with neoplastic metastases. Other predilection sites in older animals are joints with moderate to severe osteoarthrosis, especially the coxofemoral joint. The most common cause of osteomyelitis is surgical repair

Figure 2.10 Mediolateral view of the antebrachium of an 11-year-old mixed-breed dog. There is moth-eaten lysis within the diaphysis of the radius at the junction of the middle and distal thirds. Ill-defined periosteal new bone can be noted on the cranial cortex of the radius in that area. This lesion appears moderately aggressive. Histologic diagnosis: metastasis from a prostatic carcinoma.

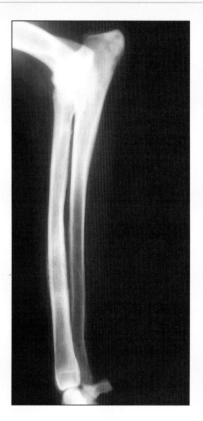

Figure 2.11 Lateral view of the thoracolumbar junction of a 12-year-old collie cross-breed dog. There is a focal, lytic lesion with well-defined margins (long arrows) within the lamina and spinous process of T13. This can be compared with the normal dorsal lamina of L1 (short arrow). Diagnosis: metastasis from a lung carcinoma.

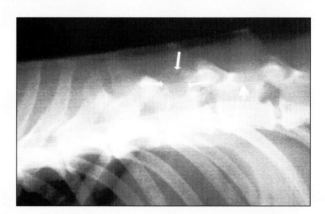

of fractures (*Figure 2.12*). Osteomyelitis may also arise as a result of direct inoculation from a bite wound, especially in cats. Such lesions are more common in the distal limbs and tail. Osteomyelitis often involves multiple bones and will cross joint spaces.

Radiographs cannot provide a histologic or cytologic diagnosis. Detection of an aggressive skeletal lesion is merely the first step in the investigation. The patient should be evaluated for the presence of systemic disease. A definitive diagnosis requires a fine-needle aspirate or biopsy of the lesion.

Figure 2.12 Mediolateral view of the antebrachium of a 6-month-old German shorthaired pointer dog. Radial and ulnar fractures have been repaired by insertion of intramedullary pins. There is mild soft tissue swelling surrounding the distal two thirds of the antebrachium. Periosteal new bone surrounds the diaphysis of the radius and ulna. At the margins of the fractures, the new bone is irregularly marginated and less well mineralized. These changes appear mildly aggressive, active, and chronic. New bone formation due to instability is usually confined to the area adjacent to the fracture. The extensive new bone formation that extends some distance from the fracture in this case indicates osteomyelitis.

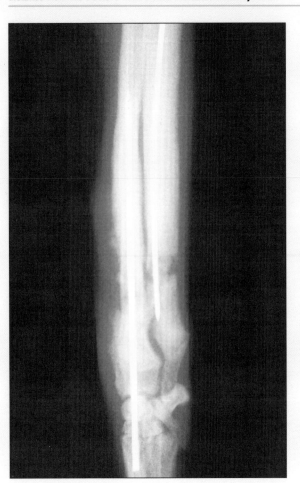

Degenerative Joint Disease (Osteoarthrosis)

Degenerative joint disease (DJD), or osteoarthrosis (OA), is a common progressive inflammatory and degenerative disease of synovial joints. DJD may occur as a primary process or occur secondary to a primary joint disease, such as osteochondrosis, surgery, trauma, or following joint sepsis. Radiographically, the first sign of DJD is the presence of soft tissue swelling. In most joints, this is not readily appreciable unless severe. In the shoulder joint and stifle joint, however, the presence of periarticular fat pads outlines the soft tissue of the joint capsule.

In the shoulder joint, a pad of fat is present caudodistal to the caudal margin of the articular surface of the proximal humerus. This may be displaced or obliterated by joint swelling. In the stifle joint, the infrapatellar fat pad fills a triangular area bordered by the patellar ligament, the cranial aspect of the proximal tibia, and the cranial aspect of the distal femur (*Figure 2.13*). Normally the soft tissues of the stifle joint are visible as a thin rim of soft tissue opacity

Figure 2.13 Mediolateral view of a normal stifle. The double-headed arrow indicates the location of the infrapatellar fat pad between the patellar ligament and the soft tissues of the stifle joint. The other arrow indicates the fat in the fascia at the caudal aspect of the stifle joint.

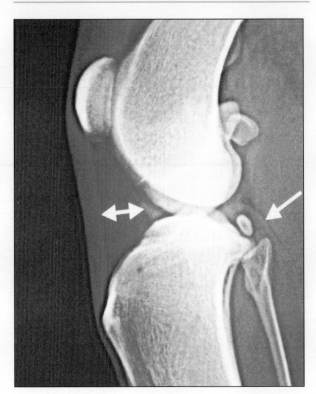

adjacent to the distal femur. Intra-articular effusion, capsular thickening, and/or periarticular edema may compress and even obliterate the fat pad. This finding is especially useful, as this swelling precedes the development of bony changes.

Periarticular osteophytes develop as a result of DJD and are new bone formations at the margins of the articular surface (*Figure 2.14*). Their size, opacity, and margination depend on the duration of the DJD. One should be familiar with the locations of osteophyte formation in specific joints. Enthetic osteophytes, or enthesiophytes, form at the site of attachment of a soft tissue structure, such as tendon, ligament, and joint capsule to bone. They may arise in response to trauma or joint instability.

Figure 2.14 Close-up ventrodorsal view of the left hip of a 7-year-old German shepherd dog. The acetabulum is shallow, and large osteophytes are present at the cranial and caudal acetabular rims and on the femoral neck. Note that the joint space is irregular. The cranial aspect of the joint space is markedly narrowed. This indicates destruction of the articular cartilage. Diagnosis: hip dysplasia, with moderate to severe degenerative joint disease.

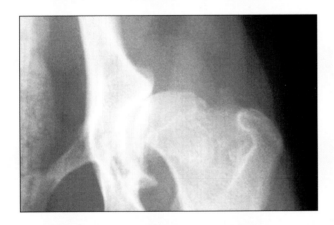

As DJD progresses, it results in irreparable injury to the articular cartilage, which may eventually be completely destroyed. Injury to the articular cartilage may result in the development of sclerosis, that is, increased opacity, of the subchondral bone. Complete or focal destruction of the articular cartilage may be appreciated on radiographs as narrowing or collapse of the joint space. Detecting joint narrowing radiographically may require that the film be obtained with the animal bearing weight on the affected joint, an approach that is not routinely performed in companion animal practice. Erosion or fracturing of the articular cartilage may also lead to the growth of so-called

subchondral cysts. These develop due to synovial fluid being pumped into fissures in the subchondral bone. They are rare in companion animals but may be seen in cases of chronic, severe, hip DJD.

Fractures and Normal Fracture Healing

Fractures may occur as a result of trauma or a defect in the bone (a pathologic fracture), such as mineral loss due to chronic renal disease or a destructive tumor. Classification systems for fractures have been described and are reviewed extensively elsewhere. In the case of traumatic fractures, at a minimum one should determine if the fracture is open or involves a joint, as these factors will determine the method of repair and the prognosis for healing. A classification system for physeal fractures has also been described, but the important thing to remember with any such injury is the possibility of premature physeal closure. If there is no history of trauma or minimal trauma, a pathologic fracture should be suspected.

Focal lesions, such as primary bone tumors or bone cysts, may cause pathologic fractures. Loss of opacity or new bone formation at the margins of a recent fracture suggests the presence of a preexisting lesion that weakened the bone. Generalized loss of bone mineral, such as occurs with nutritional or renal secondary hyperparathyroidism, may weaken the bone sufficiently to cause fractures. In such cases, there may be multiple fractures, often of different ages. Radiographs are an insensitive test of bone loss, requiring at least 70% depletion of mineral for detection. The skeleton may appear less opaque than normal, with little contrast between it and the soft tissues; and the cortices of the bones appear thin.

Primary fracture healing occurs with rigid fracture fixation, such as is achieved by a dynamic compression plate or, sometimes, an external fixator. Radiographically, it is characterized by minimal or no formation of callus. Secondary bone healing is more common and occurs when less than completely rigid internal fixation is achieved (ie, intramedullary pin), a fracture gap remains following reduction, external coaptation is used, or when no support is provided. A periosteal callus develops, initially of fibrous tissue and cartilage and, finally, bone. The callus may be quite large if the fracture is unstable during healing.

The process of bone healing is characterized radiographically as a sequence of visible changes. Recent fractures have sharply marginated, well-defined bone fragments. The first radiographic evidence of bone healing is loss of opacity and sharpness at the fracture edges. The bone at the fracture becomes necrotic due to disruption of the blood supply, creating a hypoxic, acidic environment. Osteoclasts are mobilized and resorption of the fracture ends begins, causing the fracture gap to appear wider. Formation of periosteal new bone at the edges of the fracture is the next visible change.

Mineralization is first visible radiographically at 1 to 3 weeks following injury, initially as poorly defined, hazy areas, which coalesce to form a bony callus. Eventually a trabecular pattern develops as the callus becomes more organized. This may take weeks to months and usually accompanies restoration of the endosteal and periosteal blood supplies. Finally, there is a slow remodeling of the fracture callus to allow function and restore normal or near normal strength. The time from fracture to complete healing is extremely variable, depending on the severity of the trauma, stability of fixation, degree of reduction, presence of infection, and nutritional status of the patient.

Abnormal Bone Healing

Delayed union is an intermediate stage in fracture healing and may progress either to union/malunion or to nonunion. It is defined as failure of completion of fracture healing within the expected time period for a given fracture type and/or fixation technique.

In nonunion, the fracture ends fail to unite and all healing has stopped; it may be either viable or nonviable.

Viable nonunions produce bone at the fracture ends but fail to bridge the gap. Hypertrophic nonunions have an "elephant's foot" appearance, with abundant callus and flared fracture ends (*Figure 2.15*). The fracture gap is filled with fibrocartilage, which may act as a false joint. Slightly hypertrophic nonunion is a milder form of the "elephant's foot," and oligotrophic nonunions show no evidence of callus and the fracture ends may round off. Nonviable nonunions have necrotic or poorly perfused bone segments in the fracture gap, which prevent healing. Instability and poor blood supply result in inadequate osteogenesis. Atrophic nonunion is a form of nonviable nonunion frequently encountered in the distal antebrachium of toy breed dogs. The

bones atrophy to thin points, and the fracture gap is widened (*Figure 2.16*). Malunion is defined as fracture healing with abnormal anatomic alignment of the bones.

Metabolic Bone Disease

Homeostasis of blood calcium and phosphorous levels and the metabolism of bone mineral are controlled by three major hormonal mechanisms: parathyroid hormone, calcitonin, and 1,25-dihydroxycholecalciferol. Calcium homeostasis is not only essential to the integrity of the skeleton but to the body as a whole, as calcium is an important electrolyte for many cellular functions.

The chief cells of the parathyroid glands secrete parathyroid hormone (PTH), and secretion is closely related to blood calcium levels. A fall in calcium produces a rapid rise in PTH secretion, and a rise inhibits secretion. The biologic effects of PTH are primarily on bone and kidney. PTH promotes the release of calcium from bone and decreases phosphate reabsorption. PTH is also believed to enhance the reabsorption of calcium. The C cells of the thyroid gland produce calcitonin. In bone, calcitonin prevents the release of calcium into the plasma by inhibiting the effects of PTH and promotes phosphaturia. The principal effect of 1,25-dihydroxycholecalciferol (1,25-DOHCC) is to increase intestinal absorption of calcium and phosphorus.

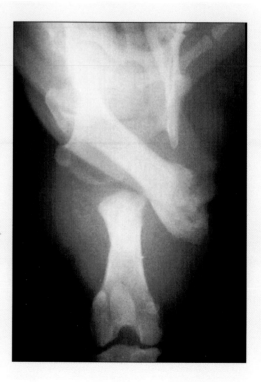

Figure 2.15 Craniocaudal view of the femur of a 4-year-old mixed-breed dog. A car had hit the dog approximately 4 months before presentation. There is a mid-diaphyseal fracture of the femur. Both the fracture ends are rounded with smoothly marginated, well-defined, well-mineralized, new bone formation. There is overriding of the fracture with proximal and lateral displacement of the distal fracture fragment. Diagnosis: hypertrophic nonunion.

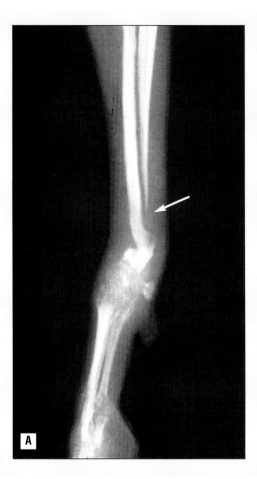

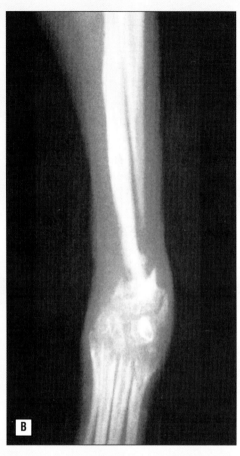

Figure 2.16 Mediolateral (A) and craniocaudal (B) views of the antebrachium of a 2-year-old Chihuahua dog. This dog had suffered radial and ulnar fractures 6 months before presentation. There is a healed malunion fracture of the distal radius with cranial angulation. The diaphysis of the ulna tapers to a point (arrow), and a large fracture gap is present. There is generalized loss of opacity in the small carpal bones and proximal metacarpals. Diagnosis: healed malunion radial fracture, atrophic nonunion ulnar fracture, and loss of bone opacity in the carpal bones due to disuse.

Renal Secondary Hyperparathyroidism

Clinical signs of renal secondary hyperparathyroidism are usually associated with the renal disease rather than skeletal lesions. Typically these include polyuria, polydipsia, vomiting, diarrhea, weight loss, anorexia, dehydration, and depression. Renal disease results in chronic hyperphosphatemia and chronic hypocalcemia, which, in turn, stimulates PTH secretion and parathyroid hyperplasia. Loss of renal tissue causes reduced production of 1,25-DOHCC, which exacerbates the hypocalcemia by preventing intestinal absorption. Calcium is resorbed from the skeleton in response to PTH secretion.

The bones of the skull are typically more severely affected, and the first radiographic signs are loss of the lamina dura and interalveolar bone around the teeth. This loss is followed by fibrous thickening and diffuse loss of mineral in the maxilla and mandibles. Thickening or widening of the muzzle may be noted on physical examination. The disease is colloquially called "rubber jaw" due to the loss of rigidity in the maxilla and mandible (*Figure 2.17*).

Figure 2.17 Lateral view of the skull of an 11-year-old mixed-breed dog. There is diffuse loss of bone mineral. Note how the teeth appear quite opaque, and the bones are almost soft tissue opacity. Diagnosis: renal secondary hyperparathyroidism.

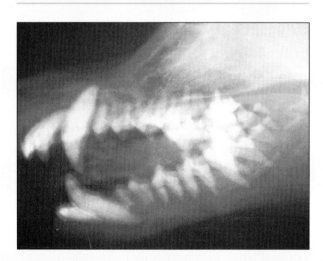

Nutritional Secondary Hyperparathyroidism

Nutritional secondary hyperparathyroidism is most commonly seen in young animals and exotic pets. It may occur because of a diet that is deficient in calcium or has a calcium/phosphorous imbalance. Clinical signs usually reflect locomotor disturbances, such as lameness, paresis, and paralysis. The pathogenetic mechanism is similar to that of renal secondary hyperparathyroidism, but the entire skeleton is uniformly affected.

Radiographs of affected animals show poor contrast between bone and soft tissues (*Figure 2.18*). The cortices of the long bones are thin and often show multiple fractures. Some of the fractures may be of the folding type. Compression fractures of the vertebrae are also common and may result in paraparesis or paraplegia. Correcting the diet causes a rapid and dramatic improvement in skeletal mineralization. Fractures usually heal quickly but deformities may persist. Vertebral fractures accompanied by neurologic deficits carry a more guarded prognosis.

Hypertrophic Osteopathy

Hypertrophic osteopathy, also known as Marie's disease, is a clinical syndrome of swelling of the extremities secondary to periosteal proliferation and edema, and painful and swollen joints. Hypertrophic osteopathy is associated with various malignancies or chronic infections of the lung or pleura or the abdominal cavity. The lesions have a characteristic appearance with well-mineralized, palisade-type new bone formation along the metaphyses and diaphyses of the long bones; the epiphyses are spared (*Figure 2.19*). New bone growth begins at the periphery, especially the metacarpal and metatarsal bones, and progresses toward the trunk.

Alternate Imaging of the Skeleton

Computed Tomography

Computed tomography and nuclear medicine are widely used in institutional and referral practice to evaluate the musculoskeletal system. Computed tomography (CT) uses x-rays to produce cross-sectional images. An x-ray tube

Figure 2.19 Mediolateral view of the antebrachium of an 11-year-old Irish setter dog. There is moderate soft tissue swelling of the antebrachium. Palisade-type new bone is notable along the metaphyses and diaphysis of the radius and ulna. This new bone is well mineralized and irregularly marginated. Notice how the epiphyses have been spared. Diagnosis: hypertrophic osteopathy. Thoracic radiographs revealed a pulmonary mass that was determined to be an adenocarcinoma.

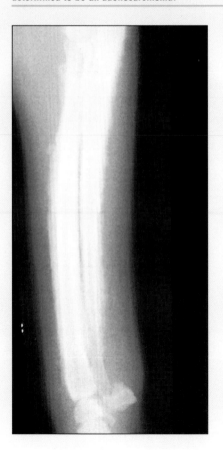

Figure 2.18 Lateral view of the thoracolumbar spine of a 5-month-old domestic shorthair cat. There is poor mineralization of all the skeletal structures. The endplates of the vertebral bodies appear very opaque in comparison with the remainder of the spine, and there is poor contrast between the soft tissues and bones. These changes indicate greater than 70% loss of bone mineral content. Diagnosis: nutritional secondary hyperparathyroidism. (The owner had been feeding a diet consisting almost entirely of raw meat.)

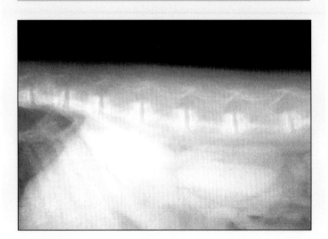

produces a thin beam that passes through the patient, and the pattern of x-rays transmitted through the patient is recorded by an array of detectors. The x-ray tube and detectors rotate around the patient while recording multiple sets of data. These data are processed by a computer and used to generate an image representing a cross-section of the body part being examined.

CT images can distinguish between different soft tissues and produce superb bone detail. Images are adjusted to maximize the contrast between the structures being evaluated. If one is interested in soft tissues, even slight differences in tissue can be seen as changes in the shade of gray in the image. When evaluating bone, the image is adjusted so that the fine structure of the bone is visible; but, by doing so, all the soft tissues appear uniformly gray with no contrast. An iodinated contrast agent is frequently administered intravenously for CT studies. Many lesions have altered vascular permeability and the small quantities of contrast agent that leak from the blood vessels produce a marked degree of lesion enhancement on CT images.

The cross-sectional images generated by CT allow evaluation of structures that may be partly or completely obscured by overlying shadows on conventional radiographs. Skull and spinal lesions are better imaged by this technique. CT is also useful for imaging joints, especially in cases of fragmentation of the medial coronoid process of the elbow and osteochondritis dissecans of the tarsus. (See Case 13, page 105.)

Nuclear Medicine

Nuclear medicine, or skeletal scintigraphy, provides a completely different perspective on skeletal disease. A short-lived radioactive agent is injected and binds to the crystal mineral matrix of the bone. This agent is selectively deposited in areas of increased skeletal turnover, so any lesion that causes bone remodeling causes increased uptake. The radioactive agent is imaged using a gamma camera. Nuclear medicine is significantly more sensitive than radiography. The images produced yield limited anatomic information but provide a map of skeletal turnover. Such lesions as degenerative joint disease, tumors, osteomyelitis, and stress fractures are detected with ease and, in some cases, long before there are radiographic changes. Nuclear medicine is an excellent tool for screening the entire skeleton, as the imaging can be done quickly and accurately. (See Case 1, page 93.)

Chapter 3: The Appendicular Skeleton

Many of the specific diseases that affect the appendicular skeleton occur in juvenile or immature animals. In diagnosing these conditions, the general principles outlined in the preceding chapter on musculoskeletal disease are used, but one must also be aware of which diseases affect specific breeds and specific joints as well as at what age they are most likely to occur.

Osteochondrosis/Osteochondritis Dissecans

Osteochondrosis/osteochondritis dissecans is a disorder of enchondral ossification, which is an important cause of lameness in young dogs. Abnormal enchondral ossification occurs and is characterized by a failure of differentiation of the chondrocytes so that the cartilage matrix is not mineralized. This impairs development of blood vessels in the area and prevents resorption of the cartilage and formation of bone. The cartilage continues to grow and becomes thickened and less resistant to mechanical stress. This cartilage relies on diffusion of nutrients from joint fluid, which cannot occur when the thickness increases, resulting in degeneration and necrosis in the basal layers. Fissures develop and may reach the joint space, undermining a flap of cartilage (osteochondritis dissecans), which in turn may give rise to free cartilage fragments that may mineralize (joint mice).

Osteochondrosis has a multifactorial etiology; genetic, nutritional, biomechanical, and endocrine factors have been implicated. Lesions are seen in large and giant breed, rapidly growing dogs, with males more commonly affected than females. Depending on the joint affected, the onset of lameness ranges from 3 to 10 months of age. The joints usually affected in dogs are the shoulder, elbow, stifle, and tarsus. Lesions are often bilateral.

Radiographic signs of osteochondrosis have common features regardless of the joint involved. These include:
- flattening of subchondral bone or widened joint space (thickening of articular cartilage),
- subchondral bone sclerosis,
- mineralized flap or osteochondral fragments ("joint mice"),
- joint effusion, and
- secondary osteoarthrosis/degenerative joint disease.

Osteochondrosis/osteochondritis dissecans affects only certain joints in dogs and specific sites within these joints as follows:
- Shoulder—caudal aspect of the humeral head (*Figure 3.1*).
- Elbow—medial distal humeral condyle (see the following discussion of "Elbow Dysplasia").
- Stifle—lateral femoral condyle and occasionally medial femoral condyle (*Figure 3.2*).
- Tarsus—medial ridge of the talus and occasionally lateral ridge of the talus.

Figure 3.1 Mediolateral view of the shoulder of a 6-month-old Labrador retriever dog. The caudal aspect of the humeral head is flattened and irregularly margined. A thin, mineralized structure (arrows) is seen adjacent to the caudal humeral head. This represents a mineralized cartilaginous flap within the joint pouch. Diagnosis: shoulder osteochondritis dissecans (OCD).

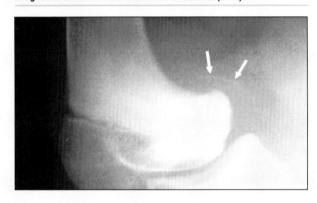

Figure 3.2 Mediolateral (A) and caudocranial (B) views of the stifle of a 6-month-old Labrador retriever dog. The joint capsule bulges cranially, compressing the infrapatellar fat pad, and caudally, displacing the fat in the fascia (arrows), indicating there is moderate to severe joint effusion and/or capsular thickening. In the caudocranial view, the distal aspect of the lateral femoral condyle is flattened. Compare the appearance of the flat articular surface of the lateral femoral condyle to the rounded normal convex outline of the medial femoral condyle. A thin, mineralized structure is notable adjacent to the caudal aspect of the femoral condyles on the mediolateral view and represents a poorly mineralized flap of cartilage (large arrow). Diagnosis: OCD of the lateral femoral condyle.

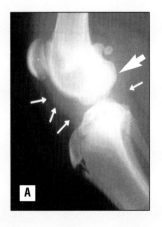
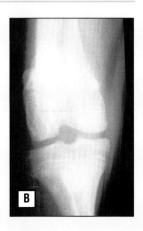

Elbow Dysplasia

Elbow dysplasia is a syndrome that comprises three conditions—fragmented coronoid process (FCP), united anconeal process (UAP), and osteochondrosis (OCD) of the distal medial humeral condyle—which may occur alone or in combination. Large and giant breeds of dogs are affected, and lameness usually occurs at 4 to 6 months of age. Bilateral involvement is common and degenerative joint disease (DJD) is an inevitable sequel to these diseases. Radiographic signs of elbow DJD include osteophytes on the proximal aspect of the anconeal process (usually the first place these are visible), radial head, medial epicondyle of the humerus, and medial coronoid process of the ulna. If there is clinical evidence of elbow lameness, then the joint should be evaluated for signs of these diseases. UAP and OCD are readily detected, but FCP may be a diagnosis of exclusion.

The anconeal process normally fuses with the body of the ulna by 16 to 20 weeks of age. Failure of fusion results in UAP and leads to joint incongruity and secondary osteoarthrosis. In addition to large breed dogs, chondrodystrophic breeds, such as basset hounds and dachshunds, can be affected. The lesion is best seen on a flexed mediolateral view of the elbow (necessary to separate the anconeal process from the medial epicondyle of the humerus). A radiolucent gap separates the anconeal process from the olecranon, and there are usually signs of secondary DJD (*Figure 3.3*).

Osteochondrosis/osteochondritis dissecans of the trochlea of the condyle of the humerus occurs in young large and giant breed dogs, especially Labrador and golden retrievers and rottweilers (*Figure 3.4*). The lesion is best seen on a craniocaudal projection of the elbow with the leg slightly supinated; this position shows a shallow concave defect in the subchondral bone of the trochlea of the humeral condyle, with or without a mineralized flap. Secondary DJD is present in longer-standing cases.

FCP is characterized by fragmentation of the medial coronoid process of the ulna, which results in osteoarthrosis (*Figure 3.5*), and is the most common developmental disease of the elbow in dogs. The diagnosis may be difficult, as one does not usually see a free or distinct fragment, and is often based on excluding other forms of elbow dysplasia, the presence of DJD in a young animal, and clinical findings. A craniocaudal projection with the leg slightly supinated may disclose a fragment or an osteophyte on the medial coronoid process. Blunting or absence of the shadow of the coronoid process, seen through the head of the radius, may be detected on the lateral view.

Figure 3.4 Craniocaudal view of the elbow of a 7-month-old Labrador retriever dog. A small, shallow, concave defect can be seen in the articular surface of the medial aspect of the humeral condyle (arrow). A small, mineralized fragment is notable within this concave defect. Diagnosis: OCD of the distal humeral condyle.

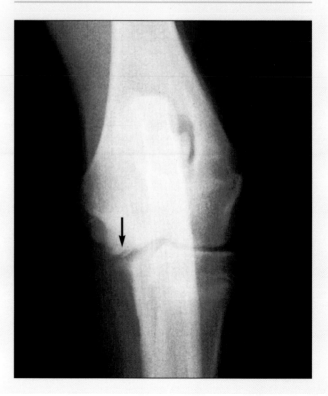

Figure 3.3 Mediolateral view of the elbow of a Great Dane dog. A radiolucent line separates the anconeal process from the body of the ulna. Diagnosis: ununited anconeal process.

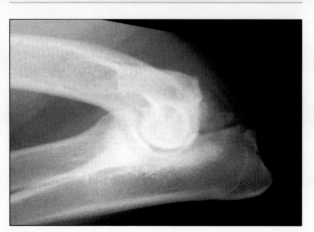

Figure 3.5 Flexed lateral (A) and craniocaudal (B) views of the elbow of a 10-month-old rottweiler dog. The long arrows indicate osteophyte formation on the anconeal process. The short arrows indicate sclerosis in the area of the anconeal process, which also represents osteophyte production. In the craniocaudal view, a moderately sized, pointed osteophyte is present on the medial coronoid process of the proximal ulna. There is no evidence of a UAP or an OCD lesion. As in most cases of fragmentation of the medial coronoid process, a distinct fragmented coronoid process cannot be identified. By eliminating UAP and OCD, FCP is the diagnosis by exclusion for a juvenile, large breed dog with DJD of the elbow. Diagnosis: elbow DJD presumed due to FCP. This diagnosis was confirmed by arthrotomy.

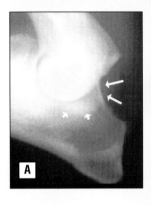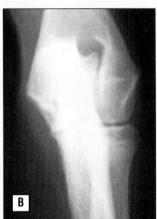

Hip Dysplasia

Hip dysplasia is a common developmental skeletal disease, which occurs in both dogs and cats but is clinically significant in medium and larger breed dogs. Hip dysplasia has a multifactorial etiology similar to that of OCD, which has not yet been fully elucidated. In immature animals, there is laxity of the coxofemoral joint, which leads to DJD and deformity of the joints. The routine ventrodorsal view of the pelvis may hide joint laxity, as extending the legs twists the joint capsule and tightens it. For this reason, most control schemes require that animals be 1 or 2 years of age before they can be certified free of hip dysplasia. The normal hip joint is a ball and socket articulation (*Figure 3.6*). The femoral head fits snugly into the acetabulum. At least 50% of the femoral head should be covered by the acetabulum. This is assessed by drawing a circle around the femoral head, the center point of which should lie medial to the dorsal acetabular rim if the joint is normal. In the cranial third of a normal joint, the articular surfaces are smooth, rounded, and parallel to each other, separated by a thin joint space. The fovea of the femoral head is flattened and can be mistaken for a pathologic change, as can the acetabular fossa.

Laxity of the hip joint is seen in immature dogs with hip dysplasia (*Figure 3.7*). If the laxity is severe, there is luxation of the hips. In less severe cases, radiographic evidence of dysplasia includes widening and incongruity of the joint space or a poorly formed, shallow acetabulum. DJD ensues, first evident as a thin line of osteophytes on the femoral neck. As the osteophytes enlarge, they fill the gap between the femoral head and the greater trochanter,

Figure 3.6 Ventrodorsal view of the pelvis of a 2-year-old collie dog. Shown are normal coxofemoral joints. Note how the femoral heads are seated in the acetabula. The dorsal rim of the acetabula can be seen through the femoral heads and is lateral to the center point of the femoral heads. Dorsal acetabular coverage is approximately 60%. The joint space is uniform in width, and no periarticular osteophytes are visible.

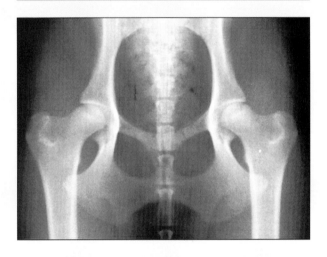

Figure 3.7 Ventrodorsal view of the pelvis of a 6-month-old mixed-breed dog. Both femoral heads are luxated; but, as yet, there is no evidence of DJD. Diagnosis: hip dysplasia.

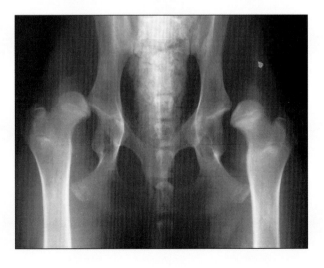

causing an apparent thickening of the femoral neck (*Figure 3.8*).

Osteophytes also develop at the cranial acetabular rim and are large if joint laxity is moderate or severe. These osteophytes may form a buttresslike structure to limit femoral head subluxation and result in the appearance of a wide, saucer-shaped acetabulum. The femoral head also remodels in response to constant instability and becomes flattened, wide, and mushroom shaped. In chronic, severe cases, the articular cartilage may be destroyed, causing narrowing of the joint space; and the subchondral bone becomes sclerotic and irregular.

Panosteitis

Panosteitis is a self-limiting inflammatory disease of the long bones and has an unknown etiopathogenesis. It is a disease that occurs in skeletally immature large and giant breed dogs, although it may occur in dogs up to 5 years of age. The affected dog presents with lameness, which may be shifting. In severe cases, the dog may be lethargic, inappetent, and febrile. There is pain on palpation of long bones, which should not be mistaken for joint-associated pain. Some dogs experience recurrent episodes. The radiographic signs lag behind the clinical signs, and films of several long bones may be required to find lesions. If the condition is acute, then radiographic signs may not have had time to develop.

The abnormalities that may be seen include increased medullary opacity, which can have a patchy or mottled appearance (*Figures 3.9 to 3.11*). In chronic cases, organized periosteal or endosteal new bone and coarsened trabeculation may be seen. Panosteitis is often overlooked or missed, as the search for a cause of lameness tends to be centered on joints. Even with radiographic evidence of joint disease, the adjacent long bones should be evaluated for panosteitis.

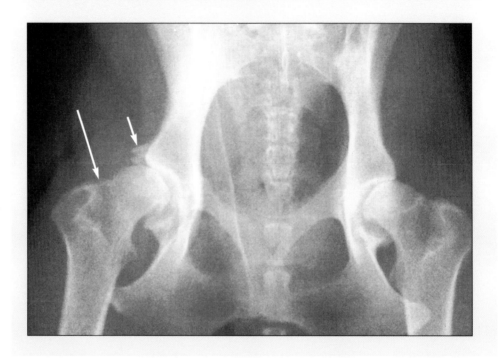

Figure 3.8 Ventrodorsal view of the pelvis of a 7-year-old mixed-breed dog. The film is slightly oblique, which can be determined by comparing the sizes of the obturator foramina. The larger foramen (in this case the left foramen) is rotated upward, away from the table. This rotation causes the acetabulum to appear deeper than it really is while making the contralateral acetabulum appear shallower. The right coxofemoral joint is moderately shallow. Large osteophytes can be noted at the cranial acetabular rim (arrow) and on the femoral neck between the greater trochanter and the femoral head (long arrow). Similar osteophyte formation is noted on the neck of the left femur. The joint space is uneven in both hip joints. Diagnosis: hip dysplasia and moderate DJD.

Hypertrophic Osteodystrophy

Hypertrophic osteodystrophy is also known as metaphyseal osteopathy and is a self-limiting and bilaterally symmetrical multifocal disease of the metaphyses affecting young, rapidly growing, large and giant breed dogs. Medium-sized dogs may also be affected but less commonly. The severity of the disease varies from short-lived mild illness to severe systemic illness. The pathogenesis is unknown, and treatment is aimed at supporting the animal. The clinical presentation is one of painful swellings at the metaphyses of the long bones, especially the distal radius, distal ulna, and distal tibia, as well as fever, lethargy, and anorexia.

In peracute cases, there may be no radiographic abnormalities; but these develop quite quickly, and changes are seen within 48 to 72 hours of the onset of clinical signs. Radiographic signs are usually bilaterally symmetrical, and the earliest change is a radiolucent line or band at the metaphyses ("double physeal line") and, occasionally, the

Figure 3.9 Mediolateral view of the elbow of a 10-month-old mixed-breed dog. There is increased opacity within the proximal ulna. Compare the appearance of the medullary cavity of the ulna, where the endosteal surface of the cortex cannot be seen, to that of the radius. Diagnosis: panosteitis.

Figure 3.10 Mediolateral view of the antebrachium of a 12-month-old Doberman pinscher dog. There is mottled increased opacity within the medullary cavity of the mid-diaphysis of the radius. Diagnosis: panosteitis.

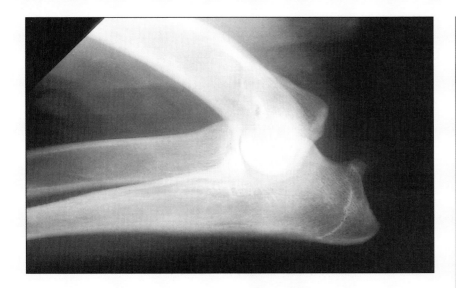

Figure 3.11 Mediolateral view of the distal humerus of a 15-month-old German shepherd dog. There is well-defined increased opacity within the medullary cavity of the distal third of the humeral diaphysis. Diagnosis: panosteitis. This lesion is well developed and chronic.

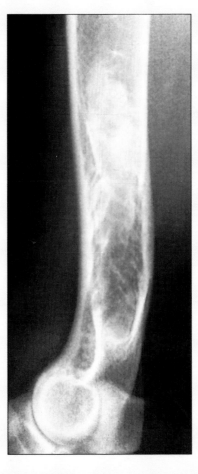

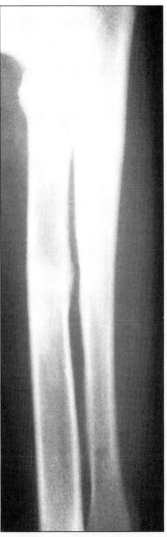

costochondral junctions, which histologically is a zone of necrosis (*Figure 3.12*). In later stages, a cuff of parosteal mineralization develops around the metaphysis as subperiosteal hemorrhage mineralizes. This cuff is gradually incorporated into the bone. A diffuse interstitial pattern may be seen if thoracic radiographs are obtained in severe cases.

Aseptic Idiopathic Necrosis of the Femoral Head in the Dog

Idiopathic necrosis of the femoral head—also known as Legg-Calvé-Perthes disease, Legg-Perthes disease, ischemic femoral head necrosis, and aseptic necrosis of the femoral head—is a degenerative condition affecting the femoral head of small and toy breed dogs. The pathogenesis is uncertain; but the disease is thought to arise in the femoral head due to multiple ischemic insults to the femoral neck, which cause necrosis of the femoral head. Occlusion of the ascending cervical arteries (the blood supply to the femoral head) causes the disease. Affected dogs present showing hindlimb lameness, with onset at 3 to 12 months.

Early changes are best seen on a "frog-leg" positioned ventrodorsal film of the pelvis. Subtle inhomogeneity and loss in bone opacity of the femoral epiphysis and widening of the joint space may be present. In later-stage cases, there is flattening of the femoral head due to osteonecrosis and a moth-eaten appearance of the femoral head and neck. In chronic cases, the femoral head is distorted and secondary osteoarthrosis develops similarly to the development of chronic severe hip dysplasia (*Figure 3.13*).

Figure 3.12 Craniocaudal (A) and mediolateral (B) views of the distal antebrachium of a 5-month-old Weimaraner dog. Mild soft tissue swelling can be seen. There are poorly defined zones of lysis parallel to the physis within the metaphyses of the distal radius and distal ulna (long arrows). In the craniocaudal view, a linear focal mineralization is seen in the soft tissues at the lateral aspect of the distal ulnar metaphysis (short arrows). Less well-developed mineralization is seen at the caudal aspect of the ulna in the mediolateral view (short arrows). Diagnosis: hypertrophic osteodystrophy.

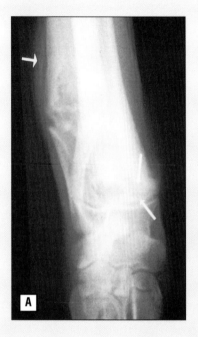
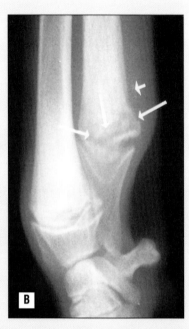

Figure 3.13 Ventrodorsal view of the pelvis of a 12-month-old Yorkshire terrier dog. There is mild subluxation of the right femoral head, which is misshapen and has an uneven opacity. Diagnosis: idiopathic aseptic necrosis of the femoral head.

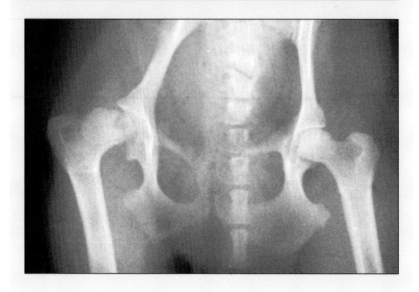

The skull and spine are complex anatomic structures and are the most challenging portion of the musculoskeletal system to interpret. In addition, there is considerable breed variation in normal skull conformation; and some breeds have anomalous vertebrae. Good positioning is essential to interpretation. Patients should always be anesthetized for skull radiographs and at least sedated for spinal radiographs. Incorporating an analgesic in the sedation protocol is recommended, as spinal disease is usually accompanied by pain. One should also be familiar with the many special projections that can be used to evaluate various parts of the skull.

Craniomandibular Osteopathy

Craniomandibular osteopathy is a disease of unknown etiology that affects immature small breed dogs, especially Scottish and West Highland white terriers. The lesions are characterized by well-mineralized, slightly irregularly to smoothly marginated, new bone formation on the caudal half of the horizontal ramus of the mandible, tympanic bullae, and the medial wall of the orbit (*Figure 4.1*). The lesions are painful in the acute phase, which often results in anorexia. The disease is self-limiting, and treatment consists of analgesics and supportive care. In some cases, however, the new bone growth is so extensive it effectively causes ankylosis of the temporomandibular joint and prevents the animal from eating. Similar lesions have been reported in large breed dogs in association with hypertrophic osteodystrophy.

Nasal Disease

Radiographic investigation of nasal disease can be frustrating. The multiple projections required to evaluate the nasal chamber and frontal sinuses are technically demanding and require general anesthesia. Changes are sometimes absent in cases where onset of signs is recent. Even in cases of severe disease, radiographs may be normal or the changes subtle and/or nonspecific. If cross-sectional imaging is available (computed tomography or magnetic resonance imaging), it should be selected over radiography. (Refer to "Computed Tomography," page 18.)

Magnetic resonance imaging (MRI) employs magnetic fields and radio frequency pulses rather than x-rays to produce images. Free protons within the body, effectively the body's water content, act as tiny magnets by virtue of their spin and electrical charge. Normally all of these tiny

Figure 4.1 Lateral (A) and dorsoventral (B) views of the skull of a 6-month-old Scottish terrier dog. A large exostosis is noted on the left tympanic bulla (arrows). This new bone is very well mineralized and well defined, with smooth margins indicating the lesion is chronic. Note the normal triangular dark air shadow of the frontal sinuses on the lateral view. Diagnosis: craniomandibular osteopathy.

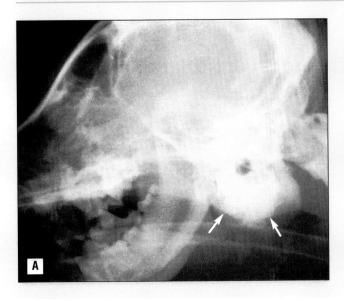
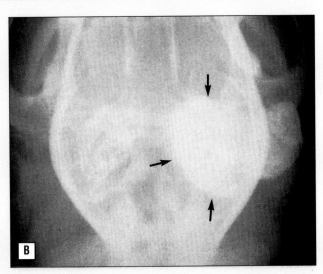

magnets are randomly oriented so there is no net magnetic field in the body. When placed in a high-strength magnetic field, however, the protons align and result in net magnetization. A short pulse of radio energy at a specific frequency disturbs this equilibrium and causes the spinning protons to wobble. The protons quickly return to the equilibrium state, and as they do so they emit radio signals. These signals are detected and processed to generate an image.

By varying the length of the radio pulse and the number of pulses, the image can be manipulated to highlight different tissue types. For example, in what are called T1-weighted images, fluid, such as cerebrospinal fluid, appears dark; but on T2-weighted images it appears quite bright (*Figure 4.2*). Contrast agents used in MRI are called paramagnetic substances. Leakage of this material from the bloodstream into abnormal tissue alters the local magnetic field and results in enhancement of the lesion.

MRI has superb soft tissue contrast and is ideally suited to evaluate such structures as the central nervous system and nasal cavity. Although MRI can be used to evaluate bone, it is more limited in that application as bone contains relatively little water and generates little signal on MRI, thus appearing dark or black.

The two major nasal diseases that may be diagnosed radiologically in the dog are neoplasia and aspergillosis. Signalment and history are of some value in determining which disease is more likely. Both diseases are rare in brachycephalic breeds. Generally, neoplasia occurs in dogs older than 7 years and nasal aspergillosis is more common in dogs younger than 7 years. These are guidelines only and exceptions do occur, however.

For descriptive purposes, the nasal chambers are divided into rostral and caudal compartments at the level of the rostral root of the fourth premolar. Neoplasms more commonly originate in the caudal portion of the nasal chamber or from the ethmoturbinates. Common radiographic findings include the presence of a soft tissue-opacity mass lesion, destruction of the nasal and ethmoid turbinate bones, and destruction of the vomer (*Figure 4.3*). Destruction of the vomer indicates that the lesion has crossed midline and that there is destruction of the nasal septum. The vomer is a small bone on the floor of the nasal chamber, however, and may be intact even if large-scale destruction of the cartilaginous nasal septum has occurred.

Soft tissue opacity in the frontal sinus is common and may be either tumor tissue or accumulated secretions due

Figure 4.2 Magnetic resonance images of the brain. A, Transverse T1-weighted image of the brain of a 12-year-old mixed breed dog that had a meningioma in the caudal fossa causing obstructive hydrocephalus. Note that both lateral ventricles are moderately dilated and that the cerebrospinal fluid is dark gray. The bones of the calvarium are black, and the subcutaneous fat is quite bright. **B,** Dorsal-plane T2-weighted image of a 6-year-old Siberian husky. This dog was evaluated for seizures, but both CT and MRI scans were normal. Note that cerebrospinal fluid and the aqueous and vitreous humors of the eye are bright. Cerebrospinal fluid can be seen surrounding the brain, and there is an appreciable difference between the gray and white matter of the cerebrum.

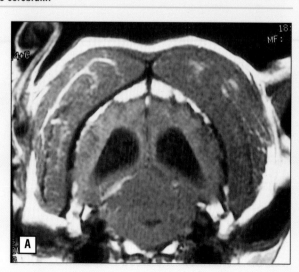

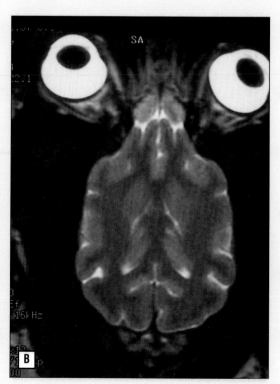

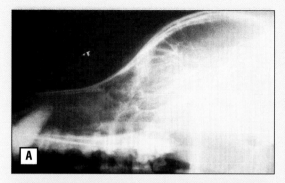

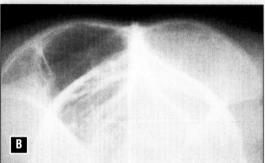

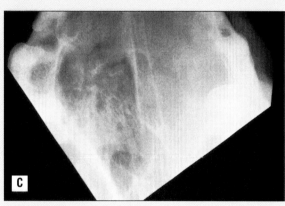

Figure 4.3 Lateral view of the skull (A); rostrocaudal view of the frontal sinuses (B); and close-up, dorsoventral, intraoral view of the nasal chamber (C) of a 12-year-old mixed-breed dog. Note the increased soft tissue opacity within the frontal sinus on the lateral view. On the rostrocaudal view, the soft tissue opacity is seen to be within the left frontal sinus and the right is normal. Note the normal, fine, linear bony structures of the turbinates in the right nasal chamber on the intraoral film. The intraoral film shows homogeneously increased soft tissue opacity within the caudal portion of the left nasal chamber and complete destruction of the turbinates. Radiographic diagnosis: soft tissue mass with turbinate destruction in the left caudal nasal chamber, most likely neoplasia. This lesion was a nasal adenocarcinoma.

to occluded drainage. Tumors may expand beyond the nasal chamber; and, if a superficial facial mass is present, tangential projections should be obtained to evaluate whether the underlying bone is intact. Canine nasal neoplasms are almost always malignant, and an aggressive pattern of bone destruction is usually seen if the tumor expands beyond the confines of the nasal chambers.

Nasal aspergillosis is also called destructive rhinitis, as the disease is characterized by destruction of the turbinates. Usually the disease begins in the rostral portion of the nasal chamber and progresses caudally. In chronic cases, it extends to involve the frontal sinuses. There may be destruction of the nasal turbinates and superimposed increased soft tissue opacity due to accumulated exudates and hemorrhage. In those cases, it is impossible to distinguish neoplasia from infection. In more chronic cases, the complete destruction of the nasal turbinates results in a hyperlucent, that is, excessively dark, appearance to the nasal chambers (*Figure 4.4*). Diffuse moth-eaten lysis of the bones of the nasal chambers and face may be seen in chronic cases.

Figure 4.4 Ventrodorsal open-mouth view of the nasal chambers of a 4-year-old pointer dog. There is increased lucency within the left nasal chamber, which appears quite black. There is complete destruction of the turbinates within the rostral and caudal portions of the left nasal chamber. Mild loss of opacity is also noted within the rostral nasal chamber on the right. Diagnosis: destructive rhinitis. Nasal aspergillosis was confirmed by endoscopy and serology.

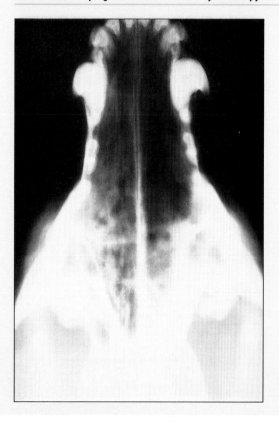

Cross-sectional techniques, such as computed tomography or magnetic resonance imaging, are far more useful than radiography for the investigation of nasal diseases (*Figures 4.5 and 4.6*). They are much more sensitive and can detect relatively small lesions. Extension of the disease beyond the nasal chamber, especially into the orbit or through the cribriform plate into the brain, can only be reliably detected by these means. Computed tomography and magnetic resonance imaging provide superior diagnostic information and better guidance for biopsy procedures, and they are essential for treatment planning for tumors. (See Case 3, page 95.)

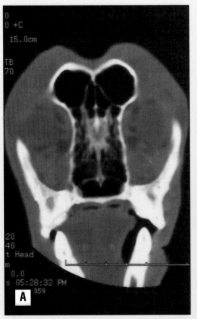

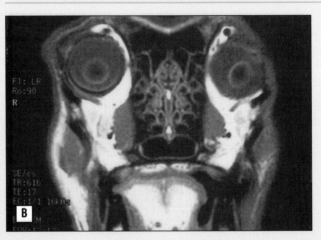

Figure 4.5 Transverse CT (A) and MR (B) images of the caudal nasal chamber of a normal 6-year-old Siberian husky. Note that the bones are quite white on the CT image. The fine scroll-like structures of the turbinates are clearly visible. This image has been adjusted to evaluate soft tissues, and fat within the orbit can be distinguished from the extra-ocular muscles. In the MR image, similar turbinate detail can be seen. The superior soft tissue imaging characteristics of this modality are evident in the ability to see the lens capsules.

Figure 4.6 Ventrodorsal open-mouth view of the nasal chamber of a 10-year-old collie-cross dog (A) and transverse (B) and dorsal plane (C) MR images at the level of the eyes of the same dog. The radiograph shows an indistinct increased soft tissue opacity in the caudal nasal chamber on the right side. There is mild loss of the normal turbinate structures in this part of the nose. The MRI scan shows an inhomogeneous mass (★), which has destroyed parts of the turbinates within the caudal portion of the nasal chamber. Note how the extent in size of the mass is significantly better defined by the MRI scan. Diagnosis: caudal nasal mass. The histologic diagnosis was carcinoma.

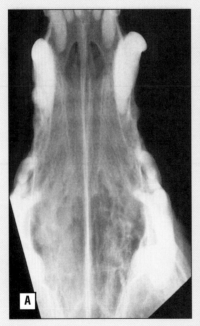

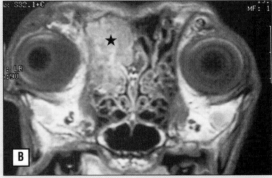

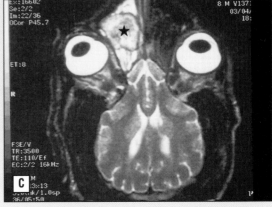

Otitis Media and Bulla Osteitis

Radiography can be used to investigate suspected middle ear disease but, as with nasal disease, is relatively insensitive; and the greater sensitivity of computed tomography and magnetic resonance imaging are preferred, if available (*Figure 4.7*). The external ear canal is assessed first. Absence of the normal tubular air shadow indicates the presence of soft tissue swelling occluding the canal, accumulated exudates, or a combination of both. Dystrophic mineralization of the cartilage of the external ear canal is a frequent abnormality in chronic otitis externa. Otitis media may be present without any radiographic change, but the presence of radiographic abnormalities generally indicates chronic and usually severe disease.

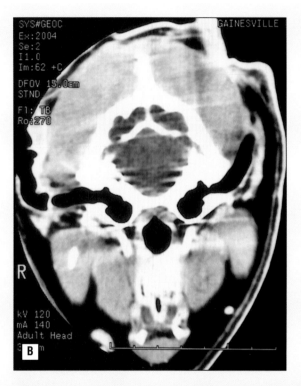

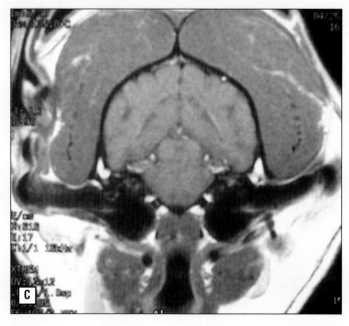

Figure 4.7 Transverse CT (A and B) and MR (C) images at the level of the tympanic bullae of a normal 6-year-old Siberian husky. A bone imaging protocol has been applied in image A, and the external ear canal is clearly seen. The fine detail of the wall of the bulla is also well demonstrated, as is the adjacent petrous temporal bone. All of the soft tissues are a uniform gray, however. The B image has been adjusted to evaluate soft tissues, and the fine detail of the bones cannot be seen as clearly. There are dark streaks within the brain in the caudal fossa; these are called beam-hardening artifacts. They occur when dense bone is imaged and render CT less suitable for evaluating the caudal fossa. The MR image (C) was obtained in a slightly different plane. Clarity of the ear structures is comparable to that of the CT scans. Note the superior image quality of the brain.

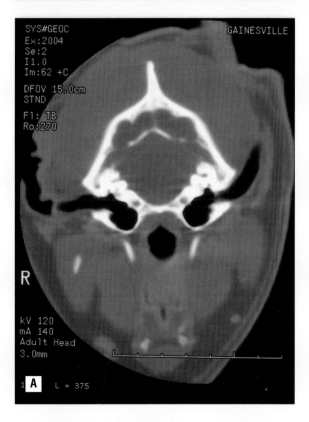

Figure 4.8 Rostrocaudal open-mouth view (A) and dorsoventral view (B) of the tympanic bullae of an 8-year-old cocker spaniel dog. There is asymmetry of the tympanic bullae on the rostrocaudal and dorsoventral films. In both views, there is increased opacity within the left tympanic bulla (long arrows), with loss of the normal air shadow. The wall of the bulla is moderately thickened. The wall of the right bulla is thin and normal and contains a normal air shadow (short arrows). Diagnosis: chronic otitis media and bulla osteitis of the left ear.

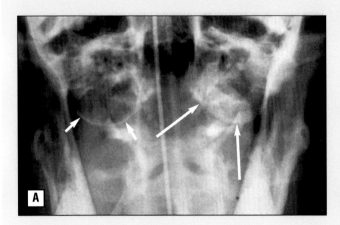 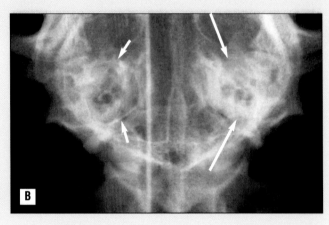

The normal air shadow of the bulla may be replaced with uniform soft tissue opacity (*Figure 4.8*). Sometimes thickening of the wall of the bulla also occurs. These changes can be assessed by comparison of left and right bullae, if the disease is not bilateral. Similar changes are seen associated with nasopharyngeal polyps in cats. These arise from the mucosa within the bulla as a sequel to viral upper respiratory tract infections. The polyp usually lies within the nasopharynx, and the cat is presented with a complaint of respiratory stridor. Neoplasia of the osseous bulla is rare but should be suspected if there is expansion of the bulla or any evidence of osteolysis.

Atlantoaxial Instability

Atlantoaxial instability or subluxation is a clinical syndrome of small and toy breed dogs. These animals may present with clinical signs as young puppies or with acute onset of signs as adults, often associated with a traumatic event. The atlantoaxial articulation allows rotation of the head around its long axis and is formed by a depression in the caudoventral aspect of the atlas and a large projection, the dens, at the cranial end of the axis.

The dens is held in place by a number of strong ligaments. Instability may arise for number of reasons. The dens is a separate center of ossification and may be hypoplastic or absent. Fracture of the dens can also occur. This may happen before skeletal maturity at the junction of the dens with the cranial epiphysis of the axis or at approximately the same level in adult dogs. Rupture of the supporting ligament of the dens can also result in instability or subluxation.

When atlantoaxial instability is suspected, a lateral survey film of the cervical spine should be obtained with minimal handling of the animal. In a well-positioned straight lateral film, the wings of the atlas are superimposed on the dens and obscure it. So if one is attempting to diagnose instability, a slightly oblique lateral view is preferred. The space between the arch of the atlas and the spinous process of the axis is small and fixed. A widened gap indicates instability (*Figure 4.9*). If support is needed, the diagnosis can be confirmed by comparing a neutral lateral film with one obtained following careful, slight ventroflexion of the neck. In a normal animal, no movement of the axis relative to the atlas is seen in such a film. Even slight widening of the gap between the arch of the atlas and the dorsal spinous process of the axis is abnormal.

Intervertebral Disk Disease

Degenerative disease of the intervertebral disks is common in middle-aged and older dogs, especially chondrodystrophic breeds. Spondylosis deformans is new bone formation around the margins of or bridging an intervertebral disk space. This new bone forms in an attempt to stabilize a degenerative or unstable disk and is commonly associated with degenerative disk disease. Spondylosis deformans is very common in middle-aged and older dogs and is almost invariably clinically insignificant.

The clinical signs associated with intervertebral disk dis-

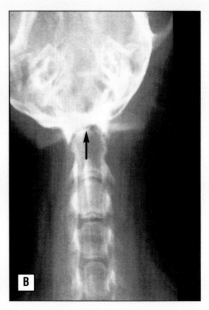

Figure 4.9 Lateral (A) and ventrodorsal (B) views of the cranial cervical spine of a 5-month-old Yorkshire terrier dog. The space between the spinous process of the axis and the arch of the atlas is widened, and there is slight malalignment of the atlantoaxial articulation on the lateral view. On the ventrodorsal view, no dens can be seen at the cranial aspect of the axis (arrow). Diagnosis: atlantoaxial subluxation.

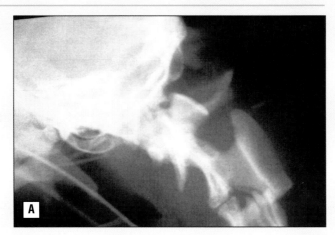

ease are variable, ranging from pain or gait abnormality to paralysis with loss of deep pain sensation. Degeneration of the disk nucleus results in loss of concussive capacity due to dehydration. In chondrodystrophic dogs, mineralization of the disk nucleus is a common event, so detecting mineralized disk nuclei is not in itself a significant finding. Degeneration of the fibers of the annulus fibrosus results in protrusion of the disk into the vertebral canal or prolapse of nuclear material into the canal if the annulus ruptures. When evaluating the spine for evidence of a disk prolapse or protrusion, one should keep in mind that some older animals may

have many such lesions and that the disks with obvious radiographic changes may not be clinically significant at the time of presentation.

The cardinal sign of disk prolapse is narrowing of the intervertebral space (*Figure 4.10*). This should be assessed by comparison of the suspect disk with the disk spaces cranial and caudal. The film must be well positioned; and only the disks in the center portion of the image should be assessed, as the x-ray beam diverges and parallax distortion causes disks at the periphery of the image to appear narrowed. If a disk is suspected to be abnormal, then a film should be taken cen-

Figure 4.10 A and B, Lateral view of the thoracolumbar spine and lateral myelogram of an 11-year-old dachshund dog. There is narrowing of the L1-2 disk space (long arrow), and the associated intervertebral foramen (short arrow) and articular facet joint space are also reduced in size in comparison to adjacent disks (A). Increased opacity is noted within the intervertebral foramen at L1-2. Note the mineralized disk nucleus at T13-L1, which is contained within the disk space. Disk mineralization is a common finding in chondrodystrophic dogs. Positive contrast agent was injected into the subarachnoid space to outline the spinal cord, a myelogram. The myelogram (B) shows marked attenuation of the contrast-filled subarachnoid space centered over the L1-2 disk, confirming the presence of spinal cord compression. Diagnosis: L1-2 intervertebral disk prolapse.

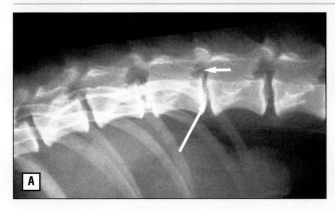
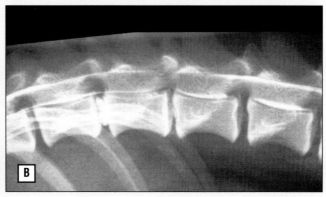

tered over it to confirm or refute this suspicion.

Along with evaluating the disk space, the intervertebral foramina and facet joint spaces should also be assessed for narrowing. A mineralized disk nucleus contained within an intact annulus appears as a well-defined, slightly ovoid object. If the annulus is weakened, then the dorsal aspect of the nucleus may appear pointed as it bulges into and through the annulus. A thin line of mineralized disk material may be seen dissecting through the annulus in some cases of disk prolapse, the so-called "toothpaste sign." Mineralized disk nucleus within the vertebral canal may cause a faint or hazy increased opacity in the intervertebral foramen or appear as a well-defined, well-mineralized structure within the vertebral canal (*Figure 4.11*). Although survey films are helpful, many dogs with disk disease have multiple lesions of varying ages and significance. Definitive localization of a cord-compressive lesion requires myelography, computed tomography, or a combination of the two.

Spinal Neoplasia

Although degenerative disk disease is the most common acquired lesion of the vertebral column, it is important to evaluate the entire structure and not to focus only on the disk spaces. Each vertebra should be assessed by two views

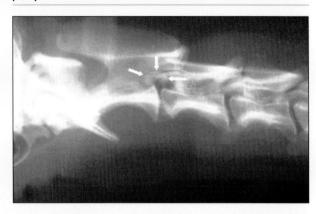

Figure 4.11 Lateral view of the cranial cervical spine of a 9-year-old beagle dog. A well-defined, ovoid, mineralized structure (arrows) is noted within the vertebral canal dorsal to the C2-3 disk space. The C2-3 disk space is moderately narrowed in comparison with the C3-4 and C4-5 disk spaces. Compare the relationship of the atlas to the axis with *Figure 4.9A and B*. Diagnosis: C2-3 disk prolapse.

for size, shape, opacity, and margination. Tumors may selectively destroy only a small part of the bone, such as a single pedicle or a transverse process (*Figure 4.12*). One should examine all the components of each vertebra in turn—endplates, ventral cortex, floor of the vertebral canal, pedicles, lamina, and facets.

Figure 4.12 Lateral (A) and ventrodorsal (B) views of the cranial lumbar spine of a 9-year-old Bernese mountain dog. There is a focal, lytic, poorly defined lesion within the second lumbar vertebra seen on the lateral film (short arrows). Also on the lateral film, note the thin line of the normal floor of the vertebral canal in L3 (long arrows), which is absent in the second lumbar vertebra. In addition, there is irregularly marginated, poorly mineralized, new bone formation along the ventral aspect of the body of L2. In the ventrodorsal view, the arrows indicate the normal left-side transverse process (L2) and normal right side pedicle of L3. The right-side transverse process and right pedicle of L2 are absent. Diagnosis: aggressive, mixed, productive and destructive lesion of the L2 vertebra. The histologic diagnosis was malignant histiocytosis.

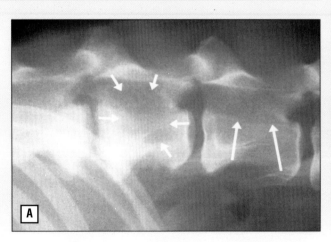

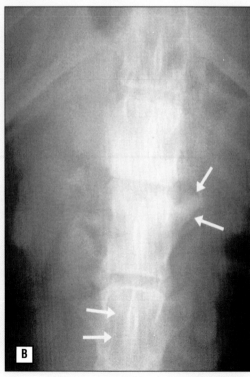

Pathologic compression fractures may be evident as a subtle foreshortening of the vertebral body. When such fractures are present, it is important to assess the opacity of the vertebra and to look for evidence of new bone formation. Traumatic compression fractures result in increased opacity as the bone mineral is compacted into a smaller volume. Pathologic compression fractures usually occur as a result of an osteolytic process, and the opacity of the fractured vertebra is equal to or less than the adjacent normal vertebrae. New bone forms within 7 to 10 days of a traumatic fracture; thus, the presence of new bone in a more recent fracture usually indicates the fracture is pathologic.

Cervical Spondylomyelopathy

Cervical spondylomyelopathy, which is commonly called wobbler syndrome, is a disease of large and giant breed dogs, especially the Doberman pinscher and the Great Dane. The disease is characterized by malformation of the canal of cervical vertebrae, which are funnel shaped (usually C5, C6, and C7), causing a narrowing of the vertebral canal at the cranial orifice. There may also be deformity of the vertebral bodies, which are more triangular in shape than normal, and instability of the disks causing malalignment and subluxation (*Figure 4.13*). The soft tissues of the disk annulus and the vertebral ligaments hypertrophy in an

Figure 4.13 Lateral view (A) of the caudal cervical spine and myelogram (B) of a 6-year-old Doberman pinscher dog. The body of C6 has an abnormal form, appearing slightly wedge shaped. The C5-6 and C6-7 disk spaces are narrowed, especially at their ventral aspect. The body of C6 is tilted dorsally, and there is mild to moderate malalignment of the spine at C5-6. The myelogram demonstrates dorsal displacement and attenuation of the ventral contrast-filled subarachnoid space, indicating a disk protrusion at C6-7 (arrow). No compression is noted at C5-6, but ventroflexed and dorsiflexed films are required to exclude compression because the lesions are often dynamic. Diagnosis: cervical spondylomyelopathy.

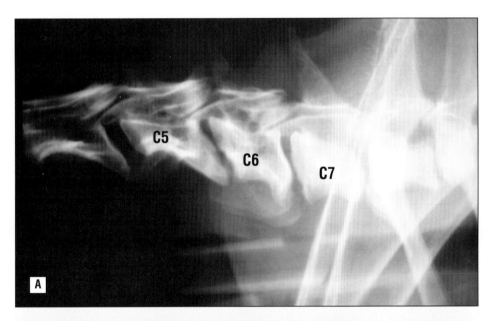

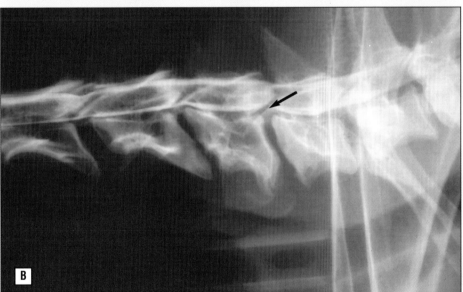

attempt to reduce the instability. This proliferative tissue is a significant component of the spinal cord compression. In middle-aged and older dogs, there is often coexisting degenerative disk disease. The cord compression is usually dynamic, that is, exacerbated by movement of the spine. Diagnosis and evaluation requires myelography.

Diskospondylitis

Diskospondylitis, or intradiskal osteomyelitis, is defined as an infection originating within the intervertebral disk space. The infection first destroys the soft tissues of the disk, and the earliest visible change is narrowing or collapse of the disk space. Lysis of the vertebral endplates occurs, resulting in an apparent widening of the disk space (*Figure 4.14*). The margins of the vertebral bodies are quite ragged and irregular, and the vertebrae may appear mildly to moderately foreshortened. In chronic cases, exuberant spondylosis deformans develops in an attempt to contain the infection and stabilize the disk.

Staphylococcus spp, *Brucella canis*, and *Aspergillus* spp are common etiologic agents. The organisms can usually be isolated from blood or urine. If a diskospondylitis lesion is detected, it is recommended that survey radiographs of the entire spine be obtained, as some cases produce multiple lesions. Radiographic progression of healing is slow.

Spondylosis deformans develops and, initially, the new bone appears active and disorganized. Complete fusion of the vertebral bodies is the desired end point.

Figure 4.14 Lateral view of the lumbar spine of an 8-year-old German shepherd dog. There is lysis of the endplates of the vertebral bodies and collapse of the intervertebral disk spaces. Moderate to severe sclerosis surrounds the disk spaces. At the L2-3 disk space, there is ill-defined lysis of the caudal endplate of L2 with a concave appearance and mild sclerosis of the adjacent vertebral body. That appearance indicates a recent lesion. There is more severe sclerosis adjacent to the lytic lesions of the other vertebral endplates indicating these lesions are chronic. Diagnosis: diskospondylitis at multiple sites. *Aspergillus* spp was cultured from the dog's urine.

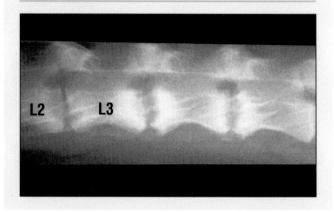

Part III

Radiology is an invaluable tool in evaluating the organs of the thorax. It is one of the quickest and easiest diagnostic tests to perform, and the air-filled lungs afford an ideal window by which to assess the heart and circulatory system. The thorax, however, is also the most intimidating body part in terms of radiographic evaluation; and many students and practitioners struggle with thoracic radiographic interpretation. By application of a systematic approach, thoracic films can be extremely rewarding (see box below).

Film Quality

Perhaps the single most overlooked factor in interpreting thoracic films is film quality. Good quality films are easier to read; and, even if one is unable to reach a diagnosis, one is more likely to get a useful report from a radiologist by sending good films.

The Normal Thorax— Helpful Rules of Thumb

Cardiac size varies depending on the breed, ranging two and one-half to three and one-half intercostal spaces wide on lateral films and one half to two thirds the width of the thorax on ventrodorsal (VD) or dorsoventral (DV) films. Deep-chested dogs are at the lower end of this range, bar-rel-chested dogs at the upper end (*Figure 5.1*). Cats should measure two to two and one-half intercostal spaces on the lateral, one half to two thirds the width of the thorax on VD/DV (*Figure 5.2*). In old cats, the heart tilts cranially, so the cardiac width should be measured perpendicular to a line from the base to the apex to compensate.

Normal lungs are relatively black, and small pulmonary vessels should be visible all the way to the periphery. Pulmonary arteries and veins should be approximately equal in size, measuring one half to equal the width of the proximal third of the fourth rib (cranial lobar vessels) or ninth rib (caudal lobar vessels) where they cross it. The cranial mediastinum should not exceed the width of the spine except in such breeds as the Boston terrier, bulldog, or pug; very obese animals; or immature animals with a normal thymus.

Systematic Evaluation

The entire film must be reviewed, even if a huge mass is found in the lung or if the heart looks normal and the films were taken because the dog had a murmur. The author has found the most reliable system is to evaluate the thorax organ by organ, structure by structure, beginning at the periphery of the film, while constantly asking oneself questions. Finally, it is always essential to ask, "What have I missed?"

GENERAL PRINCIPLES OF INTERPRETATION

- **Always obtain at least two views.** In thoracic radiology, a minimum is one lateral and a ventrodorsal or dorsoventral view. An examination consisting of both left and right laterals can be used for cases of pulmonary disease, especially for suspected metastatic neoplasia or pneumonia. Lesions in the downside lung are frequently invisible, even when quite large.
- **Use a light box,** not ceiling lights or light from a window.
- **Use exposed and developed, blackened film** to limit peripheral light, and turn off light boxes that are not in use—doing so will produce a dramatic improvement in apparent film quality.
- **Be systematic**—always.

- **Avoid distraction.** If possible, review films in a quiet location.
- **Don't jump to conclusions.** Try to separate yourself from your clinical findings and keep an open mind. This is difficult in practice, but successful detachment means you will not miss those serendipitous, but nonetheless important, lesions.
- **Conversely, use clinical data to refine your search.** For instance, if you are looking for metastases, comb the entire lung field and pay special attention to the bones, but only after looking at everything else.
- **Don't panic.** Severe or extensive pathology can be confusing or intimidating but will almost always yield a diagnosis when a systematic approach is used.

Figures 5.1 Lateral (A) and VD (B) views of a normal 2-year-old rottweiler and lateral (C) and VD (D) views of a normal 2-year-old English bulldog. Note the difference in thoracic conformation. The rottweiler has a "standard" chest conformation with a thoracic cavity that is slightly deeper than it is wide. Note the shape and size of the heart. The bulldog has a thorax that is wide, shallow, and foreshortened in the cranial-to-caudal dimension. Its heart appears relatively larger in the DV view because it lies transversely across the thorax. The cranial border of the heart is partly obscured on the lateral view, which is a frequent finding in brachycephalic breeds.

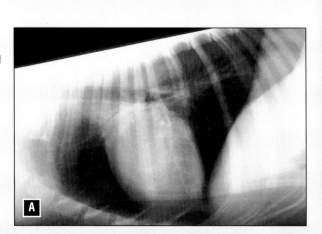

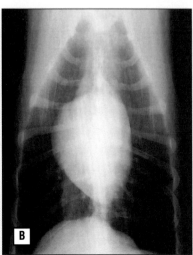

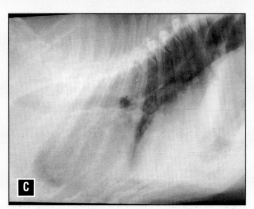

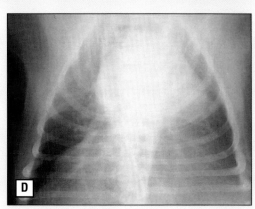

Figures 5.2 Lateral (A) and VD (B) views of the thorax of a normal 2-year-old domestic shorthair cat. The heart is slightly smaller than that of a normal dog. Note its somewhat lemonlike outline and slightly cranial tilt. A moderate amount of pericardial fat surrounds the heart on both lateral and VD views. Also note the normal appearance of the caudal lobar vessels.

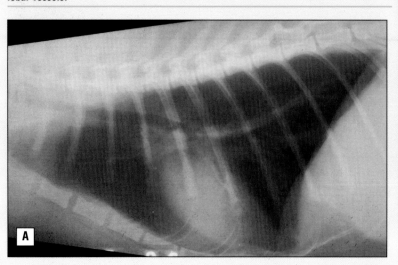

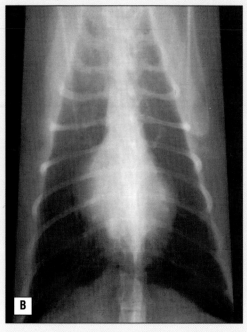

Are the soft tissues normal?

Is there a soft tissue mass or swelling?

Are the ribs normal?

Are there any rib fractures or deformities?

Is there evidence of a rib tumor?

Is the spine normal?

Is there a fracture, luxation, subluxation, diskospondylitis, tumor, septic spondylitis, or deformity?

Is there evidence of a diaphragmatic hernia?

The soft tissue and spine of the neck and cranial abdomen should also be evaluated.

The thoracic wall is often overlooked and is probably where lesions are most frequently missed. The soft tissues should be assessed for swellings or masses. These may have been found on physical examination but should still be notable on the radiographs. A diffuse swelling of the thoracic wall may cause an apparent increase in lung opacity, which could be mistaken for a real abnormality. Rib fractures can be quite difficult to detect (*Figure 5.3*). The ribs

should be examined carefully if there is a history of trauma. If a fracture is detected in an animal with no history of trauma, then the lesion should be evaluated for the possibility that it is a pathologic fracture. Rib tumors are often first noted as apparently small superficial lumps, but frequently the internal portion of the tumor is much larger. These tumors may be accompanied by pleural fluid that obscures the mass within the pleural cavity. In these cases, failure to examine the ribs results in failure to detect the tumor. These tumors are usually sarcomas and may appear lytic, productive, or both (*Figure 5.4*). Multiple lytic, productive, or mixed rib lesions indicate either skeletal metastasis or disseminated osteomyelitis. (See also sections on the "Pleural Cavity," page 51, and "The Abdominal Wall," page 67.)

Figure 5.4 Lateral (A) and VD (B) views of the thorax of an 8-year-old Dalmatian dog. A homogeneous, well-defined, round, soft tissue mass is seen in the craniodorsal thorax on the lateral film. The VD radiograph shows this to be in the right cranial hemithorax. There is leftward deviation of the trachea on the VD film and slight ventral deviation of the trachea on the lateral view. There is destruction of the proximal half of the right second rib indicating this mass originated in the thoracic wall rather in the lungs. Diagnosis: chest wall tumor. The histologic diagnosis was osteosarcoma.

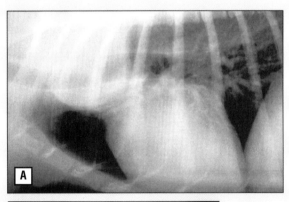

Figure 5.3 Close-up view of the right thoracic wall of a 3-year-old pug dog. There are transverse fractures of all of the ribs in this view. The fracture ends are sharp, and no evidence of new bone formation is noted. The lung lobe edges are separated from the thoracic wall by a thin band of fluid opacity. Fissure lines are seen between the right middle and caudal lung lobes. These findings indicate the presence of a small volume of fluid within the pleural cavity. This is most likely hemorrhage. Diagnosis: recent rib fractures and pleural effusion.

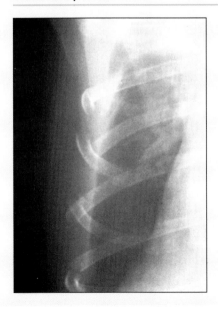

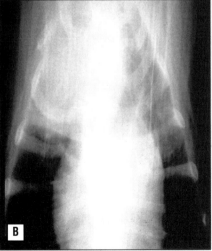

Trachea

Is the trachea normal?

Is the size of the trachea small?

If the trachea is narrowed, is the lesion focal, generalized, fixed, or dynamic?

Is there a mass or are there nodules within the trachea?

Is there a foreign body present?

Is the trachea displaced?

Usually the caudal cervical trachea is included on a thoracic radiograph. When clinical suspicion of tracheal disease exists, radiographs of the entire trachea should be obtained during inspiration and expiration. Tracheal collapse is a common clinical entity in small and toy breed dogs. Incompletely formed tracheal rings and a flaccid or redundant tracheal membrane cause narrowing of the lumen. This is usually a dynamic lesion; that is, it changes with the phase of respiration. On inspiration, there is negative pressure within the cervical portion of the trachea and it collapses or narrows (*Figure 5.5*). On expiration, positive pressure within the thorax causes narrowing or collapse of the intrathoracic trachea and, in some cases, the mainstem bronchi (*Figure 5.6*).

Uniform narrowing of the tracheal lumen is seen in tracheal hypoplasia, especially in brachycephalic breeds. Apparent uniform narrowing of the trachea is sometimes seen in dogs due to hemorrhage caused by intoxication by vitamin K antagonist rodenticides. In such cases, the air

shadow of the lumen is much smaller than the outline of the tracheal rings. A focal, fixed narrowing of the trachea is most likely a post-traumatic stricture (*Figure 5.7*). It is usually located at or just caudal to the thoracic inlet. Lesions of this kind are easily overlooked as they are small and may be partly obscured by the overlying shoulder musculature. The stenosis is the result of a healed traumatic tear of the trachea or overenthusiastic inflation of the cuff of an endotracheal tube.

Occasionally tumors arise from the tracheal mucosa and result in mass or nodule formation. Multiple nodules located at the tracheal bifurcation are caused by infestation with the worm *Osleris osleri*. Tracheal foreign bodies are

Figure 5.5 Lateral view of the trachea of a 9-year-old Yorkshire terrier dog. This is an inspiratory film. There is complete obliteration of the lumen of the caudal cervical trachea. Moderate narrowing of the intrathoracic trachea can also be noted. Diagnosis: extrathoracic tracheal collapse.

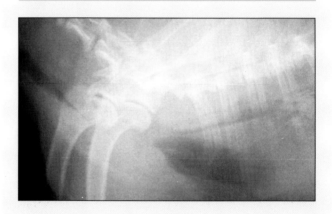

Figure 5.6 Lateral thoracic views of a 7-year-old toy poodle dog. In the inspiratory view (A), the intrathoracic trachea and mainstem bronchi are normal in diameter. On expiration (B), there is almost complete obliteration of the mainstem bronchi and moderate narrowing of the intrathoracic trachea. Diagnosis: intrathoracic tracheal and mainstem bronchi collapse.

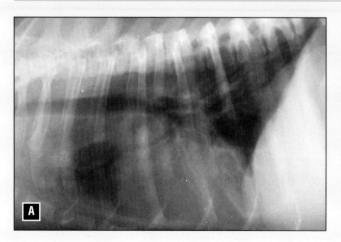

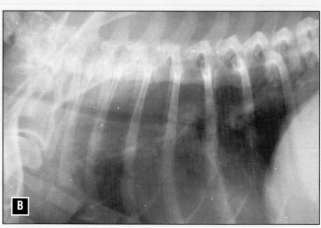

Figure 5.7 Lateral view of the cranial thorax of a 4-year-old domestic shorthair cat. There is loss of normal air shadow of the trachea in the fourth intercostal space. The lumen is narrowed to approximately 20% of the original diameter at this site by focal soft tissue swelling originating from the ventral and dorsal tracheal walls (arrows). The narrowing appears to be circumferential. Diagnosis: focal tracheal stenosis. This lesion was the result of a previous traumatic tracheal laceration.

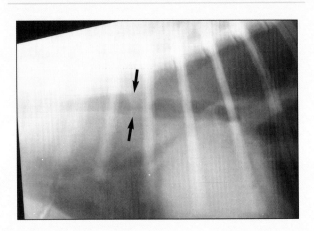

Are the bronchi normal?

Are the bronchi narrowed?

Are the bronchi displaced?

The major bronchi have walls that are thick enough to be radiographically visible in most cases, and this observation should not be mistaken for an abnormal bronchial pattern. Collapse of the mainstem bronchi during expiration is common in dogs with tracheal collapse. This is an important finding, as bronchial collapse is not amenable to surgical correction. In some cases, collapse of the bronchi can only be demonstrated by fluoroscopy. Displacement of the mainstem bronchi indicates enlargement of adjacent structures. Left atrial enlargement causes dorsal displacement of the left caudal lobar bronchus; and, rather than both bronchi being superimposed, the bronchi are split on the lateral film. Severe enlargement causes dorsal displacement of the right caudal lobar bronchus also.

On the VD or DV film, the caudal lobar bronchi are displaced laterally, resulting in a stirruplike appearance also described as the "bowlegged cowboy." Enlargement of the left atrium is most often caused by mitral endocardiosis or dilated cardiomyopathy (DCM) in dogs and hypertrophic cardiomyopathy (HCM) in cats. Similar lateral displacement of the bronchi is seen with tracheobronchial lymph node enlargement (*Figure 5.8*). On the lateral film, however, enlargement of these lymph nodes causes ventral displacement of the mainstem bronchi. Common causes of tracheobronchial lymph node enlargement include lymphoma, metastasis from primary pulmonary neoplasia, or fungal infection.

rare. Mineral opacity or metallic objects are easy to detect; but fragments of wood or leaves are more common, and their soft tissue opacity makes them more difficult to detect.

Displacement of the trachea is a very useful radiographic sign. Dorsal displacement of the cranial thoracic trachea occurs as a result of a cranial mediastinal mass. One should keep in mind that this displacement can be seen in some dogs, especially if the head is tucked down when the radiograph is taken. Before concluding a mass is present, the mediastinum must be evaluated. A heart-base mass may cause dorsal and rightward displacement of the distal trachea; generalized cardiomegaly causes dorsal displacement of the trachea. Tracheal displacement is not a reliable radiographic sign if a moderate or large volume of pleural fluid is present.

Figure 5.8 Lateral view (A) with close-up (B) and VD view (C) with close-up (D) of the thorax of an 11-year-old bull terrier dog. There is a large soft tissue mass in the region of the tracheal bifurcation. This causes ventral displacement and compression of the mainstem bronchi indicated by the arrows in the lateral close-up image (B). In the VD image, the mass can be seen lying between the caudal lobar bronchi. In the VD view, there is lateral displacement of both the caudal mainstem bronchi (arrows, D), which are moderately to severely compressed. Diagnosis: severe enlargement of the tracheobronchial lymph nodes. The histologic diagnosis was adenocarcinoma.

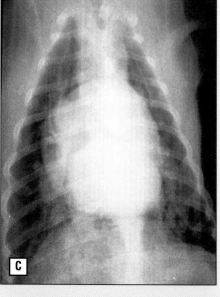

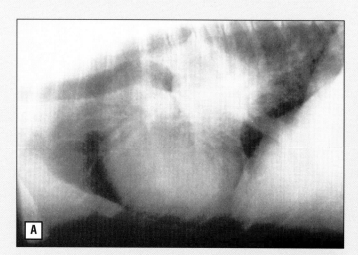

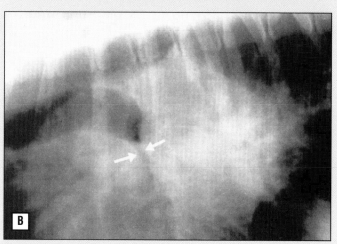

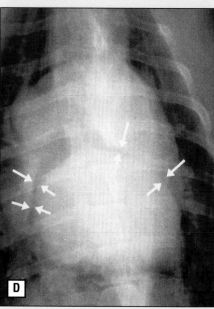

Pulmonary Parenchyma

Are the lungs normal?

Are they too dark?

Are they too light?

Which lobes are affected?

Where is the abnormality located within these lobes?

A lung that appears too dark is described as "hyperlucent." This may be a normal variant, especially in thin, deep-chested dogs (such as greyhounds) or the result of cachexia.

Abnormalities causing generalized hyperlucency include any disease that reduces the circulating volume, such as dehydration, hemorrhagic shock, or Addison's disease. Obstructive airway disease, which results in air trapping, may cause this appearance because the lesions act as one-way valves, allowing inspiration but preventing complete expiration. A common cause is feline asthma. Affected animals appear barrel chested, and the diaphragm is pushed caudally and flattened. Only one lung may appear to be affected if compensatory overinflation of one lung has occurred or if one bronchus is occluded. Focal hyperlucency may be the result of lobar emphysema, a large bullous lesion, or pulmonary thromboembolism. One should look for changes in the heart, pulmonary and great vessels, size, and overall thoracic size and shape.

A lung that is too light may indicate the presence of pathology but may also be an artifact. If the increased opacity is generalized, then it may be artifactual as a result of film that is underexposed, underdeveloped, or exposed at expiration; or the patient is severely obese. A focal or lobar increase in opacity may be the result of collapse due to prolonged recumbency or anesthesia, in addition to disease.

Having determined that the lung truly has an increased opacity, the next step is to decide which type of pattern or patterns is present. Identifying a specific pulmonary pattern is a process of elimination, as some have readily identifiable features that allow one to confirm or exclude their presence.

Alveolar Pattern

In an alveolar pattern, the air that normally fills the alveoli is replaced by fluid or displaced, in the case of atelectasis, due to collapse. The alveolar pattern has a number of specific radiographic signs that make diagnosis easier.

The air bronchogram is the gold standard radiographic sign of the alveolar pattern but is not always present. When present, the air-filled bronchus can be seen against the lung parenchyma, which contains no air and has homogenous soft tissue opacity (*Figure 5.9*). It appears as a branching dark gray line against the uniform white of the affected lung tissue.

The silhouette sign is perhaps better described as "border obliteration." If two objects of the same opacity are in contact, then the edges in contact cannot be seen. In the case of an alveolar pattern, if the portion of affected lung contacts the heart or diaphragm, the margin of those structures is obliterated. The silhouette sign can only occur if both objects are the same opacity. With lung pathology, this results only when either an alveolar pattern or a soft tissue pulmonary mass is present.

The uniformly increased opacity of an alveolar pattern causes the complete disappearance of the pulmonary vessels in the affected lung. In effect, this is another manifestation of the silhouette sign. So, if one can see vessels, the pattern is not alveolar. A common error made by novices is to interpret the large vessels on either side of a bronchus, extending from the hilus of the lung, as air bronchograms.

Bronchial Pattern

In the normal canine lung, only first- and second-generation bronchi are visible. Thickening of the bronchial

walls is seen as railroad tracks/tramlines (side-on bronchi) or doughnuts (end-on bronchi) (*Figure 5.10*). Remember that it is normal to see the larger bronchi in the hilar

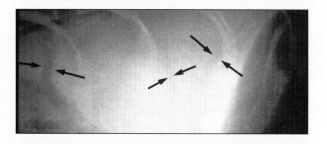

Figure 5.9 Left lateral view of the cranial thorax of a 3-year-old mixed-breed dog. There is homogeneous increased opacity within the peripheral zone of the right cranial lung lobe and middle and peripheral zones of the right middle lung lobe. Linear branching gas shadows (arrows) are noted within the affected lung. These are air bronchograms. Note that the vessels of the affected lobes are completely obscured and cannot be seen. The cranial border of the heart blends with the lung and is completely obliterated. Both of these findings are examples of a silhouette sign. The air bronchograms and silhouette signs indicate that this is an alveolar pattern. Diagnosis: bronchopneumonia.

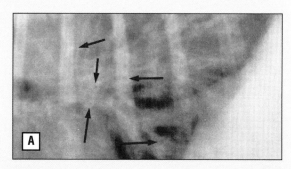

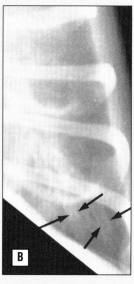

Figure 5.10 Close-up lateral (A) and VD (B) views of the thorax of a 6-year-old Siamese cat. In the lateral view, multiple ringlike or doughnut-type markings are noted within the pulmonary parenchyma (arrows). There is also a diffuse moderate increase in lung opacity. Note that pulmonary vessels can still be seen, although the smaller vascular structures are obscured by the increased opacity. In the VD view, thin, parallel, linear soft tissue structures are evident (arrows) in the periphery of the lung field. These are often referred to as "railroad tracks" or "tramlines." These findings are consistent with a bronchial pattern. Diagnosis: feline asthma.

region of the lung, but they are abnormal if the walls are thickened—this requires some experience to assess. Wall thickening has been reported as the most useful sign of bronchial disease. One should not see small bronchi especially in the middle and peripheral zones of the lungs. Bronchial mineralization should not be confused with bronchial disease. Mineralized bronchial walls are quite thin, white, and very well defined and are a normal aging change. Bronchial mineralization is usually accompanied by mineralization of the tracheal rings.

Interstitial Pattern

Interstitial patterns come in two varieties, nodular and unstructured. Nodular interstitial patterns are characterized by soft tissue nodules varying in size from 2 to 3 mm to 2 to 3 cm (when larger than 3 cm, they are typically called masses (*Figure 5.11*). Multiple, very small nodules (2 to 3 mm), often referred to as *miliary* because of the resemblance to millet seeds, may produce a snowstorm effect (*Figure 5.12*). In such cases, it can be difficult to discern a pattern; and examination of a relatively thin piece of lung, for example, overlying the ventral third of the heart or liver, is very helpful.

An unstructured interstitial pattern is present if the lung appears too light and there is nothing else to call it. This pattern is seen as a poorly defined, hazy increase in opacity, often termed a *cotton candy effect* (*Figure 5.13*). It alters the appearance of the lung by making small and medium-sized vascular structures more difficult to see. The following criteria are used to decide if a suspected unstructured interstitial pattern is real. Large vessels should be visible, although they may be difficult to discern clearly if the pattern is severe. Medium and small pulmonary vessels are obscured to a degree that depends on the severity of the pattern. If one can see small peripheral pulmonary vessels, then the suspected pattern is a phantom or the result of overzealous imagination. The bronchi may also appear more prominent

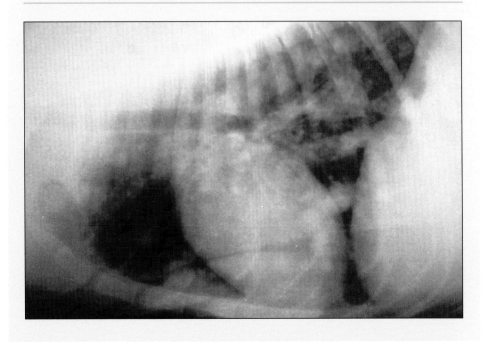

Figure 5.11 Lateral view of the thorax of a 10-year-old rottweiler dog. There are multiple, well-defined soft tissue nodules that range from 5 to 20 mm in size distributed throughout the lung parenchyma in a nodular interstitial pattern. These were metastases from a prostatic carcinoma.

against a gray lung, although not to the extent of an air bronchogram. If the lung is too gray but some vessels are still visible, it is an unstructured interstitial, rather than alveolar, pattern.

Having decided what type of pattern is present, the next step is to define the distribution of lesions. The location of lesions provides valuable clues in the differential diagnosis. Airborne or airway-associated disease may have a peribronchial or ventral distribution. Diseases that are spread by the hematogenous route usually have a diffuse distribution, sometimes more severe at the periphery. Abnormalities should be classified according to the lobes affected (some/all) and distribution within the affected areas. The lung field is divided into three concentric zones originating at the tracheal bifurcation: hilar, middle, and peripheral. Other useful descriptive observations include peribronchial, focal, or generalized distribution.

Differential Diagnosis of Pulmonary Patterns

A differential diagnosis can be refined based on pattern recognition, lesion distribution, and the presence of secondary lesions.

Figure 5.12 VD view of the right caudal lung field of a 12-year-old mixed-breed dog. There are multiple small pulmonary nodules throughout the visible lung field. These are miliary nodules, which are so numerous that the overall effect is like that of a snowstorm. In such cases, individual nodules are often easier to see at the periphery of the lung where relatively fewer lesions are super-imposed on each other. These were metastases from a splenic hemangiosarcoma.

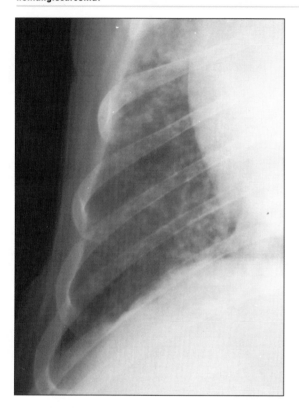

Figure 5.13 Close-up view of the caudodorsal thorax. There is a diffuse increase in soft tissue opacity. This reduces the visibility of the normal pulmonary vasculature but does not completely obscure the larger vessels. The pattern is not characterized by nodules, doughnuts, or railroad tracks and is therefore considered an unstructured interstitial pattern. The diagnosis was pulmonary infiltrate with eosinophilia due to heartworm infestation.

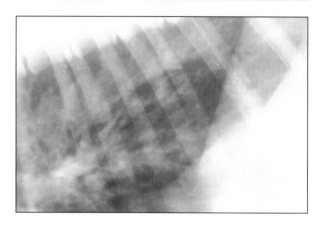

Figure 5.14 VD view of the thorax of a 4-year-old mixed-breed dog presented after an automobile accident. There is homogeneous increased soft tissue opacity within the caudal subsegment of the left cranial lung lobe. This results in obliteration of part of the outline of the left side of the heart indicating that the pattern is alveolar. Diagnosis: traumatic contusion.

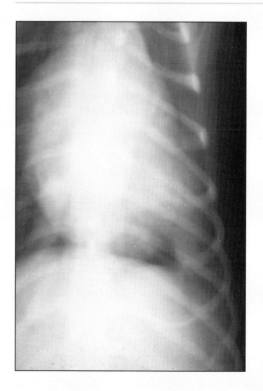

Assessing an Alveolar Pattern

The alveolar pattern can occur because of pneumonia, hemorrhage, edema, atelectasis, or neoplasia. Regardless of the type of disease that causes the pattern, its appearance is much the same. Distribution within the lung and the presence of secondary signs are most useful in refining the differentials in the diagnostic list.

Blood

Hemorrhage may be due either to trauma (*Figure 5.14*) or a coagulopathy. The distribution is random and can be quite extensive, especially in such diseases as disseminated intravascular coagulation (DIC). Look for signs, such as rib fractures and pleural air, to confirm trauma.

Pneumonia

Bronchopneumonia typically has a ventral distribution, affecting the peripheral and middle zones of the right middle, right cranial, and left cranial lung lobes (*Figure 5.15*). The lesions begin at the periphery of the lung lobes and extend to the hilus with increasing severity. Complete alveolar opacification of the right middle lung lobe is a common finding. Aspiration pneumonia has a similar lobar distribution but may have a peribronchial location, especially if the lesion is acute. One should look for evidence of esophageal dysfunction, which supports a diagnosis of aspiration pneumonia. Remember that esophageal dilation may be seen in severe pneumonia accompanied by severe dyspnea and will resolve if the pulmonary lesions can be successfully treated. If severe pneumonia is present, one should refrain from diagnosing a megaesophagus until the animal's dyspnea has resolved. Hematogenous pneumonia is uncommon and tends to have a patchy random distribution.

Edema

Edema is classified according to the immediate cause as cardiogenic, the result of left-sided heart failure, or noncardiogenic from any other cause. Noncardiogenic pulmonary edema is distributed in the middle and peripheral zones of the caudal lung lobes (*Figure 5.16*). When severe, it may

Figure 5.15 Right (A) and left (B) lateral views and a VD view (C) of the thorax of a springer spaniel dog. This homogeneous soft tissue opacity within the right cranial and middle lung lobes obliterates the right border of the heart. In the left lateral view, air bronchograms are visible within the middle and peripheral portions of the lung lobes indicating the presence of an alveolar pattern. Note that no abnormalities are evident on the right lateral film, as quite substantial abnormalities may be invisible if in the downside lung when taking lateral views. Both left and right lateral views should be obtained in cases of suspected pneumonia. There is a mediastinal shift with the heart displaced toward the right body wall. Diagnosis: bronchopneumonia. *Author's Note*: Bronchopneumonia is the most likely diagnosis based on the lung pattern, which lung lobes are abnormal, and the distribution within these lobes. The presence of the mediastinal shift indicates that there is loss of volume in the affected lobes, suggesting this lesion was chronic. The degree of volume loss, however, is insufficient to account for the increased opacity. Hemorrhage should also be considered in the differential diagnosis.

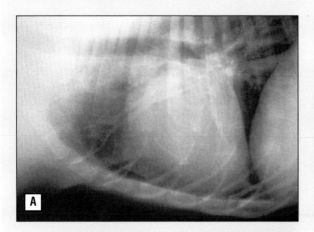

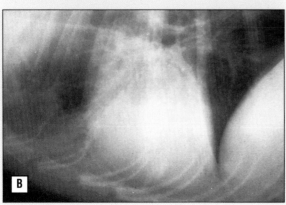

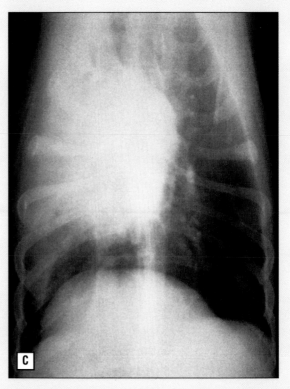

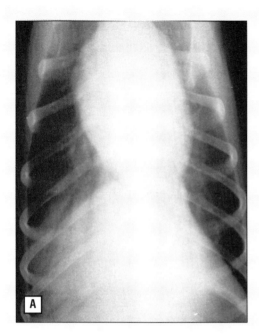

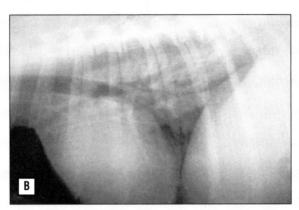

Figure 5.16 VD (A) and lateral (B) views of the thorax of a dog presented after multiple seizures. There is homogeneous increased soft tissue opacity in the middle and peripheral zones of the right caudal lung lobe. An air bronchogram is seen within this affected portion of lung in the VD view. In the lateral view, this portion of lung obliterates the outline of the crus of the diaphragm indicating an alveolar pattern. Based on the type of pattern and the location, noncardiogenic edema is considered most likely. Diagnosis: noncardiogenic edema due to status epilepticus.

extend to the hilus, resulting in an almost complete "white-out." The cranial lobes are usually spared. Causes include electric shock, status epilepticus, cranial trauma, near drowning/strangulation, and severe airway occlusion. Noncardiogenic pulmonary edema usually responds poorly to diuretic therapy.

Cardiogenic pulmonary edema is the result of left-sided heart failure. In dogs with mitral endocardiosis, it begins in the hilar region of the caudal lung lobes and extends to the periphery (*Figure 5.17*). Initially it may appear as an interstitial pattern, which coalesces to form an alveolar pattern. In dogs with DCM, a more widespread pattern is often seen in fulminant cardiac failure. The edema may be distributed throughout the lung with a peribronchial, perivascular, or random, patchy distribution rather than hilar distribution. In cats with left-sided heart failure, a similar random or patchy pattern may be seen. In cases of endocardiosis and congenital heart disease, pulmonary edema is usually accompanied by cardiac changes, such as left atrial and ventricular enlargement and pulmonary venous congestion. Similar findings can be seen in cases of DCM in dogs and HCM in cats; but, in some cases of peracute failure, there may be minimal or no change in the overall size and shape of the heart. The response to aggressive diuresis is often dramatic with complete or almost complete resolution of edema within 12 to 24 hours.

Atelectasis

Alveolar patterns are usually considered in terms of flooding the lung with a fluid and displacing air; but they can be the result of collapse, so the affected area should be assessed for any reduction in size (*Figure 5.18*). A radiographic sign, which may indicate volume loss, is the mediastinal shift; that is, the heart is pulled toward the area of increased opacity. Air bronchograms in collapsed lungs may show bronchi that appear parallel rather than diverging. Volume reduction and the presence of alveolar fluid can be combined, such as in pneumothorax with lobar collapse and contusion. The key question in determining whether an alveolar pattern is due to atelectasis or flooding is whether the increase in opacity is compatible with the reduction in volume or greater than would be expected. In other words, is one dealing with volume loss alone or is there another process too? An alveolar pattern that is solely the result of atelectasis requires an 80% or greater reduction in lung volume.

Neoplasia

Primary or metastatic pulmonary neoplasia that presents as an alveolar pattern is rare. The distribution may mimic the appearance of any of the diseases just described or be entirely random (*Figure 5.19*). This differential should be considered with alveolar patterns that have unusual or atypical distributions or that resemble one of the more common causes but fail to respond to appropriate therapy.

Figure 5.17 Lateral films of the thorax of a 3-year-old Doberman pinscher dog obtained at presentation (A) and at 12 (B) and 24 (C) hours after treatment. The trachea is displaced dorsally and runs parallel to the thoracic spine. The caudal border of the heart cannot be seen on the lateral view due to increased soft tissue opacity. Increased lung opacity also causes obliteration of the outline of the cupola of the diaphragm. Pulmonary vessels cannot be seen in the hilar region of the affected lung. This is an alveolar pattern. The cranial lung lobes and the periphery of the caudal lobes appear normal. On the second film, obtained 12 hours after diuretic therapy had commenced, the pulmonary opacity has decreased and the heart and diaphragm can be seen. A moderate, hazy, unstructured interstitial pattern persists. On the film obtained 24 hours after treatment, there has been complete resolution of the pulmonary pattern. Diagnosis: alveolar pattern with perihilar distribution and severe cardiomegaly consistent with cardiogenic pulmonary edema due to dilated cardiomyopathy. The edema resolved quickly in response to treatment.

Figure 5.18 VD view of a 3-year-old mixed-breed dog that had been hit by a car a few hours previously. Gas can be seen outlining the lateral border of all the lung lobes in both the left and the right hemithoraxes. There is homogeneous increased soft tissue opacity within the lung lobes, and the left border of the heart blends with the affected lung. The increased pulmonary opacity is too great to be accounted for by the relatively small reduction in lung volume caused by the pneumothorax. This indicates the presence of a second process, which in this case is most likely a contusion due to trauma. Diagnosis: pneumothorax, partial lung atelectasis, and contusion.

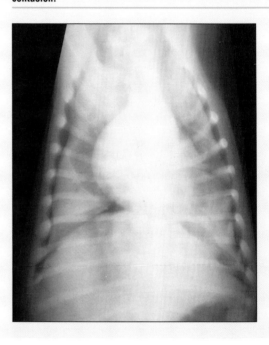

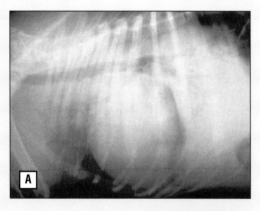

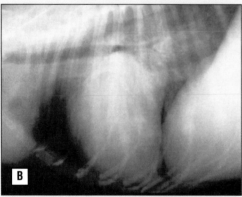

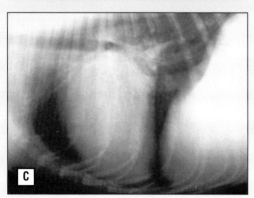

Figure 5.19 Lateral view of the thorax of an 11-year-old cocker spaniel dog. There is homogeneous increased soft tissue opacity in the cranioventral lung field. Multiple air bronchograms are seen within these lung lobes. The cranial border of the heart is partly obscured. This is an alveolar pattern. The location of the lesion is typical of bronchopneumonia or aspiration pneumonia. Neither disease correlated with the clinical presentation, however; and the dog did not respond to treatment. Histologic diagnosis: pulmonary lymphoma.

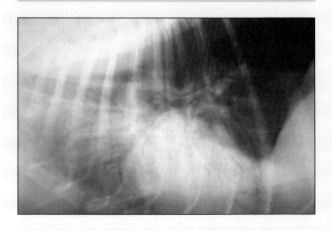

Bronchial Pattern

A bronchial pattern indicates airway disease, which may have an allergic, infectious, or inflammatory cause. Radiology is quite insensitive when diagnosing bronchial disease. In cats, asthma is the most common diagnosis. Heartworm infestation in dogs and cats may provoke an allergic response, pulmonary infiltrate with eosinophilia, which is seen as either a bronchial or unstructured interstitial pattern or a mix of both. Although heartworm disease is the most common cause of pulmonary infiltrate with eosinophilia, it occurs sporadically from other causes. A dramatic resolution of the radiographic changes may be seen after 48 to 72 hours of treatment with corticosteroids.

Nodular Interstitial Pattern

The principal differentials associated with a nodular interstitial pattern are metastatic neoplasia or disseminated fungal disease. Other rule-outs include hematogenous pneumonia, abscesses, granulomas, and parasitic lesions (such as *Toxoplasma* spp and *Paragonimus* spp).

Unstructured Interstitial Pattern

There are a myriad possible diagnoses linked to the unstructured interstitial pattern, including fibrosis, neoplasia (lymphoma, primary lung tumors, and metastases), allergic lung disease/pulmonary infiltrate with eosinophilia (often associated with heartworm disease), interstitial pneumonia (viral, early fungal, early or resolving bacterial), interstitial edema, poisoning (alpha-napthylthiourea), hemorrhage, inhalational injury, uremia, and feline infectious peritonitis. This pattern is probably the least helpful radiographic finding, and additional tests are usually required to determine its significance. Remember, it may also be caused by artifacts or any disease process that reduces the pulmonary volume, such as pleural effusion. An important consideration is that an unstructured interstitial pattern may represent disease in transition. Such a pattern is commonly seen with developing or resolving edema or bronchopneumonia or in the transition between a normal and an affected lung with these diseases.

Pleural Cavity

- Is the pleural cavity normal?
- Is there pleural fluid?
- Is there a pleural or extrapleural mass?
- Is there pleural air?

Radiographic signs associated with the presence of pleural fluid vary with the volume present and the particular view obtained (*Figure 5.20*). A film obtained with the

Figure 5.20 Lateral (A), VD (B), and DV (C) views of the thorax of a 9-year-old golden retriever dog. In the lateral view, there is dorsal retraction of the ventral border of the lung. The outline of the heart and cupola of the diaphragm cannot be seen. In the VD view, the heart can be seen outlined by the lungs. There is retraction of the lungs from the thoracic wall, and fluid opacity can be seen in the fissures between the lung lobes and separating the lungs from the thoracic wall. On the DV film, the heart and cupola of the diaphragm are completely obscured. There is a fissure line between the right caudal and middle lung lobes. Diagnosis: moderate-volume pleural effusion.

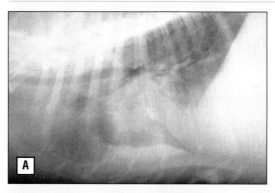

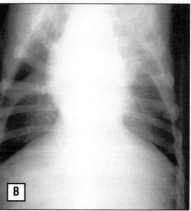

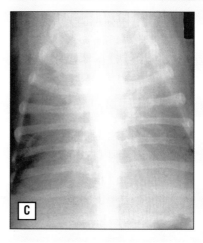

patient in sternal recumbency (DV view) is most sensitive, as fluid tends to pool in the ventral thorax and surround the heart, partly or completely obliterating the outline. On VD films, the fluid tends to pool left or right of midline in the caudodorsal thorax; and, if only a small volume is present, it will not be detected. If a large or moderate volume of pleural fluid is suspected, then the patient should not be placed in dorsal recumbency because that position results in severe exacerbation of any respiratory compromise. If evaluation of the heart is necessary, however, a VD film is required, as even a small volume of fluid will obscure the outline in the DV projection. This can be obtained after drainage of the pleural fluid.

Several changes may indicate the presence of pleural fluid. Pleural fissure lines are fluid opacity lines in the divisions between the lung lobes. One should not mistake the border of a rib for a fissure line on the VD or DV film. Pleural fissure lines are curved with the concave side facing caudally; the concave surface of the ribs faces cranially. The lung margins are retracted, that is, separated from the thoracic wall by soft tissue opacity, and the tips of the lung lobes may be rounded. Rounding is more common with chronic effusions.

The pleural fluid partially or completely obscures the cardiac and diaphragmatic outlines, which is a manifestation of the silhouette sign (see previous discussion under "Alveolar Pattern," page 45). There is a dramatic change in this appearance between DV and VD films. Pleural fluid causes a diffuse increase in opacity in the thorax, which should not be mistaken for pulmonary pathology. The pleural fluid contributes to increased background opacity and causes some degree of atelectasis, which causes the lungs to appear gray. Decisions about pulmonary pathology are best reserved until after drainage of the fluid.

Possible causes of pleural fluid include right-sided heart failure, hypoproteinemia, hemorrhage, neoplasia, infection, inflammation, pancreatitis, thoracic duct rupture, and diaphragmatic rupture. The thorax should be examined for evidence of cardiac disease, trauma, or neoplasia. Asymmetric fluid distribution or fluid that remains fixed in position warrants closer scrutiny. The ribs and thoracic wall should be examined to ensure a tumor has not been overlooked if fluid is asymmetrically distributed. The possibility of an incarcerated diaphragmatic hernia containing liver, spleen, or part of the gastrointestinal tract should also be considered.

Trapped fluid or unilateral fluid accumulation is usually the result of an inflammatory or infectious process. Pyothorax,

especially in cats, may be unilateral (Refer to *Figure 5.23.*) The mediastinum in cats and dogs is complete but permeable but may be sealed by an inflammatory effusion. Common causes of unilateral pleural effusion include pyothorax, chylothorax, and neoplasia. Fixed pockets of fluid can occur if adhesions develop between the parietal and visceral pleura, trapping the fluid in place. Ultimately, a sample of fluid must be obtained for analysis to further the diagnostic process.

Pleural Air

Pneumothorax is relatively easy to diagnose if the volume is large but can be overlooked if only a small volume of air or gas is present (*Figure 5.21*). Care should be taken not to confuse skin folds with lung margins, leading to an erroneous diagnosis. Skin folds extend beyond the borders of the pleural cavity, and pulmonary vessels will cross these lines but not the borders of collapsed lung. If in doubt, a horizontal beam lateral or VD/DV view will confirm or exclude a pneumothorax. Radiographic signs may include the following:

❏ an overall hyperlucent thorax;
❏ elevation of the heart from the sternum;
❏ retraction of the lung margins, which are outlined by air;
❏ collapsed, small, leaflike lung lobes, which appear quite opaque; and
❏ absence of any pulmonary markings at the periphery of the thorax.

A tension pneumothorax is a life-threatening emergency in which a tear in the lung acts as a one-way valve and breathing causes air to be pumped into the pleural space, progressively collapsing the lungs. Radiographic signs include an overexpanded hyperlucent thorax, collapsed very small lungs, and caudal displacement and tenting of the diaphragm. A tension pneumothorax is sometimes unilateral, and a marked mediastinal shift may be noted.

Pleural Masses

Masses arising from the thoracic wall and pleura are frequently accompanied by moderate- to large-volume effusions that obscure the tumor until thoracocentesis has been performed. Films should be evaluated for the following radiographic findings:

❏ Pleural fluid
❏ A mass with an extrapleural sign (Masses that arise from the parietal pleura or chest wall have a broad base of attachment and blend gradually with the wall of the thorax. This is referred to as the extrapleural sign.)
❏ Osteodestructive or osteoproductive changes on the ribs

Figure 5.21 Lateral (A), DV (B), and horizontal-beam VD (C) views of the thorax of a 2-year-old mixed-breed dog. The heart is separated from the sternum and displaced dorsally by a large gas bubble. On the lateral film, the dorsal border of both the caudal lung lobes is outlined by air. Pulmonary markings are not seen in the caudodorsal periphery or ventral periphery of the thoracic cavity. This finding indicates there is a pneumothorax. On the DV film, gas can be seen outlining the left caudal lung lobe. The heart is shifted toward the right thoracic wall. Air bronchograms are seen within the left caudal lung lobe, which is of homogeneous soft tissue opacity, and within the right middle lung lobe and right cranial lung lobe, which obliterate the right border of the heart. These abnormalities indicate the presence of an alveolar pattern. On the horizontal-beam VD view of the thorax, the pleural cavity is filled with gas and devoid of any pulmonary markings. Diagnosis: traumatic pneumothorax with pulmonary contusions.

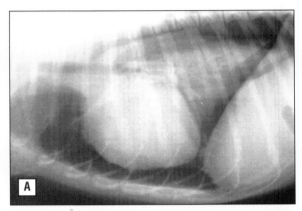

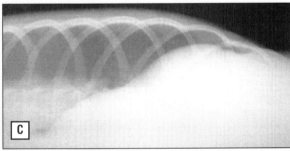

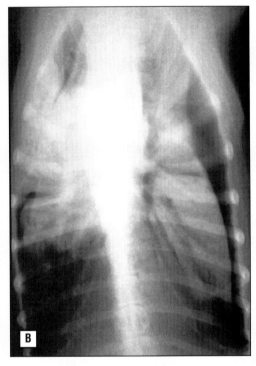

Mediastinum

Is the mediastinum normal?

Is there a mediastinal mass or fluid?

Is there mediastinal air?

Is there a mediastinal shift?

The mediastinum is formed by the reflection of the two pleural sacs. Major structures contained within the mediastinum include the thymus, lymph nodes, trachea and bronchi, esophagus, and pericardial sac. Mediastinal abnormalities that are evident radiographically are the presence of air, a mass or masses, fluid, or a mediastinal shift.

Pneumomediastinum arises due to puncture of any of the air-containing structures within the mediastinum or an external penetrating wound. It may lead to a pneumothorax but cannot happen as the result of a pneumothorax. The key to diagnosing a pneumomediastinum is the ability to see soft tissue structures, which are normally radiographically invisible, within it (*Figure 5.22*). These include:

- ☐ Both the outer and inner margins of the tracheal wall
- ☐ The entire thoracic aorta
- ☐ The great vessels of the cranial mediastinum and the azygos vein
- ☐ The longus colli muscles
- ☐ The esophagus

Mediastinal gas may extend cranially into the fascial planes of the neck and then to the subcutis, causing subcutaneous emphysema. Caudally, gas may dissect along the aorta into the retroperitoneal space.

Mediastinal tumors usually arise from the thymus or lymph nodes, ectopic thyroid tissue, or connective tissues. Mediastinal fluid may accumulate due to the presence of a mass, hemorrhage, or mediastinitis, which is usually secondary to esophageal perforation.

Figure 5.22 Lateral view of the cranial thorax of a greyhound dog. Note that both the inner and outer margins of the dorsal and ventral tracheal walls are clearly visible. A number of large, tubular, soft tissue opacity structures are also visible in the cranial thorax ventral to the trachea. These are some of the large vessels located in the cranial mediastinum and are normally invisible radiographically. Diagnosis: pneumomediastinum.

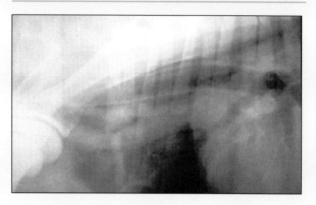

Radiographic signs of a mass or fluid include:

❏ Increased overall opacity on the lateral film

❏ Tracheal elevation

❏ Caudal displacement of the tracheal bifurcation from its normal location at the fifth intercostal space

❏ Widening of the cranial mediastinum to exceed the width of the spine on the VD or DV film (except in brachycephalic breeds)

❏ Blurring or obliteration of the cranial border of the heart

Mediastinal masses are usually accompanied by pleural fluid, which makes diagnosis difficult. Dorsal deviation of the trachea in the presence of a moderate or greater volume of pleural fluid cannot be used to infer the presence of a mediastinal mass. Repeating radiographs following thoracocentesis is helpful. Positional films may be more useful for evaluating the cranial mediastinum. An erect horizontal-beam DV or VD film is preferred. This should cause the pleural fluid to drain to the caudal thorax and the lungs to outline the lateral margins of the cranial mediastinum quite clearly.

An alternative technique is to perform a cranial venacavogram. A large-bore catheter is placed in either jugular vein, and a bolus of water-soluble iodinated contrast agent (400 to 800 mg iodine/kg) is injected as quickly as possible. A mass will cause dorsal displacement, compression, and distortion of the cranial vena cava. The vena cava should also be evaluated for the presence of intraluminal abnormalities. Within the contrast, filling defects that have a consistent appearance on multiple films suggest thrombus formation or vascular invasion by tumor. A crude assessment of cardiac size may also be made by this technique.

A mediastinal shift is really a pleural or pulmonary abnormality (*Figure 5.23*). It may occur either due to volume loss or increased volume in one hemithorax resulting in pulling or pushing of the heart to one side. The lungs should be evaluated for evidence of a mass, overinflation, or volume loss and the pleural space for air, a mass, and/or fluid. A shift occurs within minutes if the animal is anesthetized. A common cause of mediastinal shift is prolonged lateral recumbency for any reason.

Figure 5.23 VD view of the thorax of a cat. There is homogeneous soft tissue opacification of the right hemithorax, and no normal lung is present. Possible causes for this include a mass or unilateral pleural effusion due to or accompanied by an inflammatory process. The heart is displaced leftward and touches the left thoracic wall, a mediastinal shift. The left lung appears normal. Diagnosis: unilateral pleural effusion. This was found to be a pyothorax by thoracocentesis.

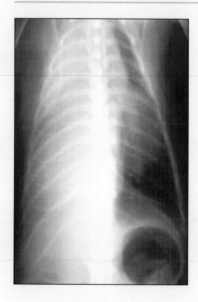

Esophagus

Is the esophagus normal?

Is the esophagus dilated?

Is there an esophageal foreign body?

Is the esophagus perforated?

The normal esophagus is radiographically invisible. Many normal animals have a short, thin, linear gas shadow within the esophagus just cranial to the tracheal bifurcation. This should only be regarded as abnormal if it persists unchanged on multiple films. Heavy sedation and anesthesia frequently cause esophageal dilation, so megaesophagus can only be diagnosed in conscious animals. Dilation of the cranial thoracic esophagus may result in a ventral and rightward displacement of the trachea. The apposed esophageal and tracheal walls are seen as a soft tissue stripe if the esophagus is gas filled and may be confused with a pneumomediastinum, but the stripe is thicker than the tracheal stripe. The walls of the caudal esophagus are outlined by luminal gas as two, thin, soft tissue stripes converging on the esophageal hiatus of the diaphragm (*Figure 5.24*).

Figure 5.24 Lateral thorax. There is uniform moderate gaseous dilation of the thoracic esophagus. Note the combined tracheal and esophageal wall, which forms a soft tissue stripe. This should not be confused with gas within the mediastinum, which outlines the walls of the trachea. The caudal thoracic esophagus is seen as two, thin, soft tissue lines converging on the esophageal hiatus of the diaphragm. Diagnosis: generalized megaesophagus.

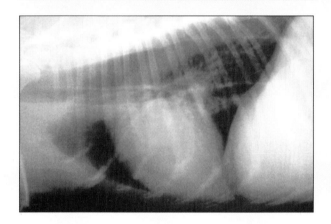

A fluid-filled, dilated esophagus does not usually have distinct margins and appears as an increased opacity in the caudodorsal thorax on the lateral film. A VD or DV view confirms the increased opacity is on the midline and prevents confusion with pulmonary pathology. It is important to distinguish segmental from generalized megaesophagus. Dilation of the esophagus cranial to the heart base is consistent with a vascular ring anomaly in immature animals. Acquired segmental megaesophagus is rare but may occur as the result of stricture formation.

Generalized megaesophagus is diagnosed if the entire esophagus is dilated. It can be congenital or acquired. Acquired generalized megaesophagus may be due to myasthenia gravis, neurologic or muscular disease, or endocrinopathies but is commonly idiopathic. It may be accompanied by aspiration pneumonia. One must carefully scrutinize the lungs for evidence of pneumonia if evidence of esophageal dysfunction is seen. Animals with severe pul-

monary disease and dyspnea may exhibit esophageal dilation due to aerophagia, however, so the presence of esophageal disease can only be accurately assessed when the dyspnea has resolved.

Esophageal foreign bodies are more commonly seen in dogs and only rarely in cats. The common sites for objects to become trapped are the thoracic inlet, heart base, and esophageal hiatus. In cats, foreign bodies may be trapped at the cricopharyngeal sphincter. Bones are easy to identify, but soft tissue-opacity objects are often overlooked, especially as owners can confuse vomition and regurgitation and the clinician's attention may be focused on the abdomen. The esophagus is usually dilated cranial to the lesions and gas may outline the foreign object. The mediastinum should be carefully evaluated for evidence of an esophageal perforation. Perforation results in mediastinitis, which is seen as a periesophageal accumulation of fluid and mediastinal gas.

The Heart

Radiology is both sensitive and insensitive, specific and nonspecific, in diagnosing cardiac disease. This may seem contradictory but one must keep in mind that it is impossible to see inside the heart, and specific changes in the cardiac chambers are extrapolated from relatively nonspecific changes in the overall size and shape of the heart. Radiology is most limited in the diagnosis of congenital heart disease and rather more useful for acquired cardiac disease. Although a disease-specific diagnosis may not be made, valuable information about the severity of cardiac changes, degree of heart failure, and response to therapy can be obtained from radiographs. Echocardiography or cardiac ultrasound can be used to assess internal cardiac structures and to quantify function.

Radiographic Assessment of Cardiac Disease

Where is the cardiac apex?
Is the overall cardiac size normal, reduced, or enlarged?
Are any specific chambers or great vessels enlarged?
Are the pulmonary vessels normal or enlarged?
Is the lung parenchyma normal?
Is there evidence of pulmonary edema?
Is there pleural fluid, hepatosplenomegaly, or ascites?
Are there sufficient data to make a diagnosis, or are additional tests indicated?

Cardiac Apex

The apex is the best external cardiac landmark by which to distinguish the left and right sides. Locating the apex is necessary to determine if the left or right side of the heart is enlarged (*Figure 5.25*). Severe left-sided cardiomegaly may cause rightward displacement of the apex on VD or DV films and mimic the appearance of right-sided cardiomegaly. On lateral films, right-sided cardiomegaly may lift the apex off the sternum. On VD films, leftward deviation of the apex may occur with right-sided cardiomegaly.

Cardiac Size

The appearance of a normal heart varies considerably with breed and conformation in dogs and with age in cats, and so do changes associated with enlargement. (Refer to "The Normal Thorax—Helpful Rules of Thumb," page 39.) For example, a heart that is three and one-half intercostal spaces wide on a lateral radiograph would be normal in a golden retriever but enlarged in a Doberman pinscher.

Reduced cardiac size is usually the result of a depleted circulating volume (*Figure 5.26*). Dehydration, hemorrhage, and Addison's disease are common causes. Microcardia may

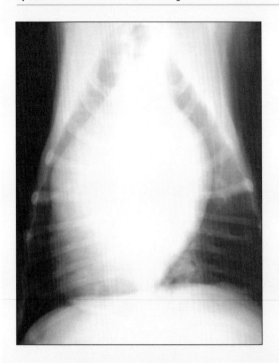

Figure 5.25 VD view of the thorax of a 4-year-old boxer dog. There is severe generalized enlargement of the heart. Note that the cardiac apex has shifted to the right side of the thorax. This creates the impression of predominantly right-sided cardiomegaly, but the apical shift indicates left-sided enlargement.

Figure 5.26 Lateral (A) and VD (B) views of the thorax of a German shepherd dog presented for weakness, vomiting, and polydipsia. In the lateral view, the heart measures two intercostal spaces wide, is lifted from the sternum by a pad of mediastinal fat, and is shorter than normal. In the VD view, the heart is small, measuring less than one third the width of the thorax. The pulmonary vessels are small and difficult to see. The lung fields are dark and uniformly hyperlucent. Diagnosis: microcardia and pulmonary underperfusion. The dog was found to have Addison's disease.

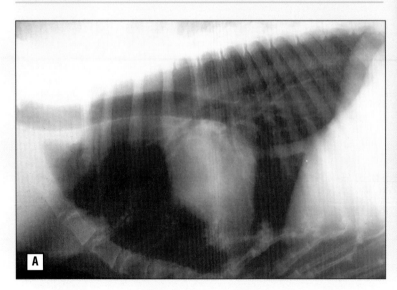

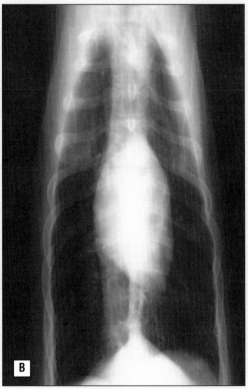

or may not be accompanied by a hyperlucent appearance of the lung and small pulmonary vessels.

Specific cardiac chambers and great vessels cannot be identified as such on radiographs but form a specific portion of the cardiac outline (*Figure 5.27*). The outline of the heart is treated as a clock face, and bulges or bumps are described based on the clock analogy.

Specific Cardiac Chamber or Structure Enlargement

Left atrial enlargement in dogs is seen as a triangular bulge at the caudodorsal aspect of the heart on the lateral film (*Figure 5.28*). In cats, the enlarged left atrium appears as a rounded bulge in the same location, altering the normal lemonlike shape of the heart to kidney bean shaped. Left atrial enlargement causes elevation and sometimes compression of the left caudal-stem bronchus and, if severe, the right also. On the VD film, the enlarged left atrium spreads the mainstem bronchi (the "bowlegged cowboy" sign) and may result in a double edge at the caudal border of the heart silhouette (6 o'clock). In severe enlargement, the left atrial appendage is seen as a bulge on the left lateral border of the heart (3 o'clock).

Left ventricular enlargement results in straightening of the caudal cardiac border on the lateral film and an elon-gated heart on the VD film. Also on the VD film, the heart border on the left side bulges and is closer to the thoracic wall than normal. The cardiac apex may be shifted to the right, creating the impression of right cardiomegaly, so before deciding if an enlargement is left or right sided, one should always locate the apex. Left ventricular hypertrophy is usually concentric (hypertrophic cardiomyopathy, aortic stenosis) and may produce no radiographic change in the size and shape of the heart unless the left atrium is enlarged or myocardial failure has occurred, resulting in ventricular dilation.

Right atrial enlargement is rare as a discrete change, with the exception of cases of feline hypertrophic cardiomyopathy. It is seen as expansion and rounding of the cranial cardiac border just ventral to the trachea on the lateral film and a bulge in the right cranial heart border on the VD film (9 to 10 o'clock).

Right ventricular enlargement results in rounding and cranial expansion of the cranial cardiac border on the lateral film and rounding of the right cardiac border, which is closer to the thoracic wall than normal on the VD film (*Figure 5.29*). In some cases, this produces the reverse-D appearance on VD or DV radiographs. On left lateral radiographs, the cardiac apex may be rounded and lifted from the sternum.

Figure 5.27 Lateral (A) and VD (B) views of the thorax of a normal dog. The arrows and numerals indicate the clock-face analogy used to describe the location of cardiac structures on both the VD and lateral films. The locations of the cardiac chambers and great vessels within the cardiac silhouette are indicated. AO = aorta, LA = left atrium, LV = left ventricle, RV = right ventricle, RA = right atrium, MPA = main pulmonary artery, LAA = left atrial appendage.

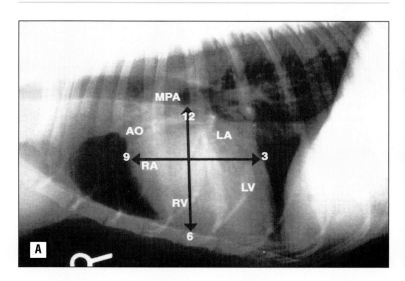

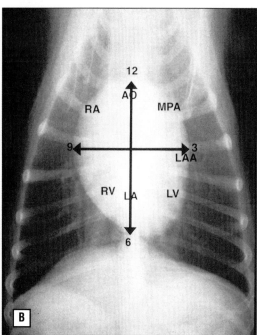

Figure 5.28 Lateral (A) and VD (B) views of the thorax of a 14-year-old toy poodle. There is severe dorsal displacement of the trachea. The heart is widened, measuring four and one-half intercostal spaces on the lateral film and over two thirds the width of the thorax in the VD view. These changes indicate severe, generalized enlargement of the heart. A triangular bulge is noted at the caudodorsal aspect of the heart on the lateral film, representing a severely enlarged left atrium. This bulge causes extreme dorsal displacement of the mainstem bronchi. The enlarged left atrium is seen as increased soft tissue opacity between the two mainstem bronchi at the caudal aspect of the heart on the VD view. The lungs are normal, and there is no evidence of cardiogenic edema. Diagnosis: generalized severe cardiomegaly with severe left atrial enlargement. Mitral valve endocardiosis and incompetence was confirmed on echocardiography.

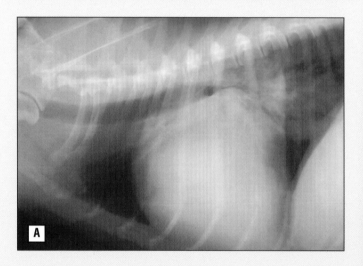

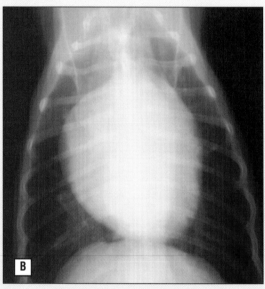

Figure 5.29 VD (A) and lateral (B) views of the thorax of a 1-year-old mixed-breed dog. The right cardiac border is rounded and expanded on the VD view, and the heart has a reversed-D type appearance. On the lateral film, the cranial cardiac border is rounded and the heart is wider than normal, measuring almost four intercostal spaces. The cardiac apex is elevated from the sternum in the lateral view. Diagnosis: moderate right-sided cardiomegaly. Echocardiography revealed tricuspid valve dysplasia.

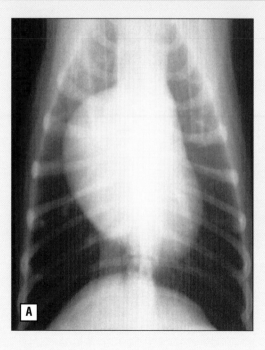

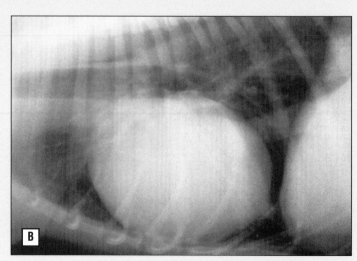

Aortic enlargement is seen as a bulge at the cranial aspect of the heart , which blends with the cranial mediastinum on the lateral and a rounded "cap" on the cranial border of the heart on the midline (12 o'clock) of the VD view (*Figure 5.30*).

An enlarged main pulmonary artery can be seen as an increased opacity just cranial to the tracheal bifurcation on the lateral film when enlarged and as a bulge at the left cranial border of the heart (1 to 2 o'clock) on the VD (*Figure 5.31*).

The size of the caudal vena cava varies considerably with the phases of the cardiac and respiratory cycles but does not exceed the diameter of the descending aorta.

Figure 5.30 VD (A) and lateral (B) films of the thorax of a golden retriever dog. On the lateral film, the heart is widened, measuring almost four intercostal spaces. There is a bulge at the cranial aspect of the heart ventral to the trachea. In the VD view, the heart is elongated with a bulge of the cranial aspect at approximately the 12 o'clock position. The heart is also widened with a rounded left border. The lungs are normal. Diagnosis: enlargement of the aortic arch and mild cardiomegaly. Echocardiography confirmed an aortic stenosis.

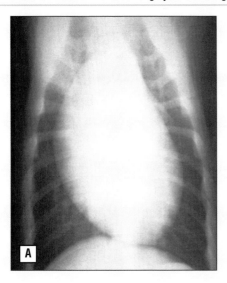

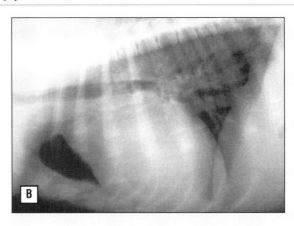

Figure 5.31 VD (A) and lateral (B) films of the thorax of 1-year-old Pomeranian dog. On the lateral film, there is rounding and expansion of the cranial cardiac border. The heart measures four intercostal spaces wide. There is mild dorsal elevation of the trachea, and the caudal vena cava is distended. On the VD film, the heart is widened, measuring almost 80% the width of the thorax. The apex is displaced toward the left thoracic wall. The right cardiac border is rounded and almost touches the right thoracic wall. This gives the heart a reversed-D type appearance. There is a bulge at the 1 o'clock position in the area of the main pulmonary artery. Diagnosis: severe right-sided cardiomegaly with main pulmonary artery bulge. A pulmonic stenosis was confirmed by echocardiography.

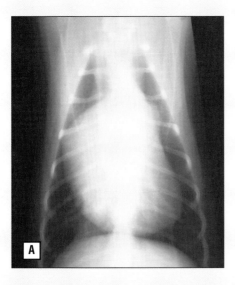

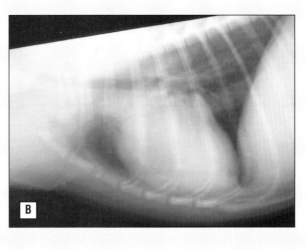

Pulmonary Vessels

Normal pulmonary arteries and veins should be approximately the same size. The cranial lobar vessels are assessed on a lateral film, where the artery is the more cranial and dorsal of the pair (*Figure 5.32*). The caudal lobar vessels are assessed on a VD, or preferably DV, film where the artery is the lateral vessel and the vein lies medially. An objective assessment of size is made by comparing the cranial lobar vessels to the fourth rib and the caudal lobar vessels to the ninth rib where they cross it. Normal vessels should be equal to or smaller than the width of the proximal third of the corresponding rib. In some cases, especially congenital shunt lesions, there may be an increase in number of radiographically visible pulmonary vessels rather than enlargement of the hilar and mid-zone portions of the vessels. In such cases, examination of the periphery and mid-zones reveals an increased number of small vascular markings or a moderate to severe unstructured or reticular (honeycomblike) interstitial pattern.

Cardiac Failure Syndromes

Left-sided heart failure occurs with volume or pressure overload of the left side of the heart. Failure causes a sequence of events beginning with pulmonary venous congestion, interstitial pulmonary edema, and eventually alveolar edema (*Figure 5.33*).

Right-sided heart failure occurs with volume or pressure overload of the right side of the heart. This leads to systemic venous congestion and pleural effusion, a small amount of pericardial effusion, hepatosplenomegaly, and ascites.

Differential Diagnosis of Cardiac Disease

Formulating a differential diagnosis is simplified by considering heart disease as either acquired or congenital. Generally, animals with signs of cardiac disease and under 5 years of age are more likely to have a congenital lesion.

Figure 5.33 Lateral (A) and VD (B) views of the thorax of a 3-month-old springer spaniel dog. On the lateral view, there is severe, generalized enlargement of the heart. This is evidenced by dorsal displacement of the trachea and widening of the heart, which measured over six intercostal spaces. Increased pulmonary soft tissue opacity partly obscures the caudal cardiac border. In the VD view, the heart is partly obscured by increased pulmonary opacity. A bulge is noted in the 12 to 1 o'clock position on the cardiac outline (arrow). The lateral border of this bulge blends with the descending thoracic aorta. Air bronchograms are noted within the hilar and middle zones of the right caudal lung lobe, and the right caudal border of the heart is obscured indicating the presence of an alveolar pattern. Diagnosis: severe cardiomegaly with aortic enlargement and left-sided heart failure with alveolar pulmonary edema. A patent ductus arteriosus was found on echocardiography.

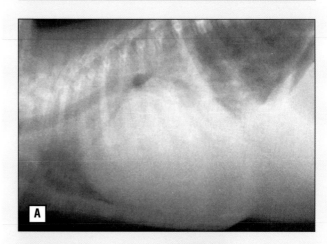

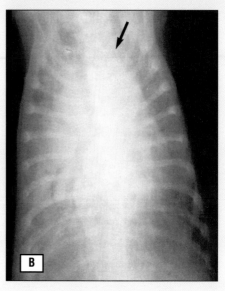

Figure 5.32 Lateral thorax of a normal dog. The cranial lobar arteries and veins are labeled.

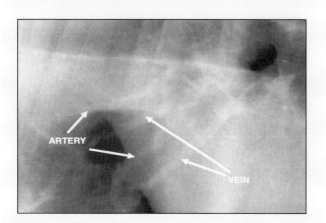

Acquired diseases, such as DCM, HCM, and heartworm disease occur in young animals, however.

Congenital cardiac disease may be classified into four major categories:

- Valvular stenotic lesions
- Valvular incompetence lesions
- Shunting lesions
- Complex lesions

Stenotic lesions most commonly affect the aortic or pulmonic valves. The outflow is narrowed at the valve (pulmonic stenosis), outflow tract (aortic stenosis), or distal to the valve. The narrowing causes increased resistance to ventricular output, resulting in concentric myocardial hypertrophy. Hypertrophy may cause little alteration of the size and shape of the left ventricle. Eventually myocardial failure develops and ventricular enlargement occurs. Hypertrophy of the right ventricle causes a rounded bulging right cardiac border on both lateral and VD films.

The high-speed jet of blood pushed through the stenosis results in turbulence, which causes dilation of the artery just distal to the lesion. A main pulmonary artery dilation is best seen on the VD or DV film at the left cranial aspect of the heart shadow (1 to 2 o'clock). Moderate or severe pulmonic stenosis causes a reduction in size of the pulmonary vessels. An aortic dilation is seen as a bulge on the cranial aspect of the heart on the lateral VD films (12 o'clock). If severe, it creates the impression of an elongated cardiac shadow on the VD or DV film.

Valvular incompetence occurs due to dysplasia and most commonly affects the atrioventricular valves. This is a common anomaly in cats and may affect either or both of the mitral or tricuspid valves. Moderate to severe atrial enlargement develops due to regurgitation of blood from the ventricle during systole. Myocardial failure ensues, and severe generalized cardiomegaly is seen radiographically. The lesions are usually severe, and significant cardiomegaly and failure occur in animals that are quite young.

Shunting lesions are the result of a persistence of a portion of the fetal circulation (patent ductus arteriosus) or maldevelopment of cardiac structures (atrial and ventricular septal defects). Flow through the shunt is from left to right unless severe pulmonary hypertension exists. The radiographic changes in the heart are variable and nonspecific.

Patent ductus arteriosus lesions may cause enlargement of the aortic arch, the main pulmonary artery, and the left atrium and, in severe atrial enlargement, the left atrial appendage. If there is enlargement of the aorta, main pulmonary artery, and left atrial appendage, then the three bulges are referred to as the "three-knuckle sign" on the VD or DV radiograph. Each aspect has been described individually. More commonly only one or both of the great arteries is enlarged. Septal defects may exhibit no radiographic abnormalities if the shunt is small or there are nonspecific changes. The best indicator of the presence of a shunt lesion is pulmonary overcirculation seen as enlargement of both pulmonary arteries and veins, an increased number of small vascular markings, and a diffuse unstructured interstitial pattern.

Complex lesions are quite challenging and are usually not amenable to diagnosis from survey radiographs. One of the more common lesions is the tetralogy of Fallot, which is a combination of pulmonic stenosis, right ventricular hypertrophy, ventricular septal defect, and overriding aorta. This combination of lesions can result in quite variable radiographic signs, depending on the severity of the anomalies. It is principally of interest because the radiographic appearance may mimic an uncomplicated pulmonic stenosis.

Differential Diagnosis of Acquired Cardiac Disease

When evaluating radiographs for suspected acquired cardiac disease, the signalment of the patient is very helpful. Valvular incompetence due to endocardiosis is most commonly a clinically significant lesion in older toy and small breed dogs. Both atrioventricular valves are affected, but the mitral valve lesion is the one that typically produces clinical signs. As valvular incompetence worsens, left atrial enlargement develops (*Figure 5.34*). Due to pressure on the left caudal lobar bronchus, this enlargement may cause a cough at night before any radiographic signs of failure are seen. The disease progresses to left ventricular dilation as the myocardium fails, and pulmonary venous congestion and edema are seen in decompensated cases. Cardiogenic pulmonary edema due to mitral endocardiosis is first visible in the hilar zone of the caudal lung lobes and spreads to the periphery. Rarely, edema may affect the right caudal lung lobe only. Tricuspid endocardiosis seldom causes purely right-sided cardiac failure, but this is seen in late-stage, left-sided disease.

Acquired left-sided cardiac disease in large and giant breed dogs is usually caused by DCM. The heart size may

Figure 5.34 Lateral (A) and VD (B) films of the thorax of a 12-year-old Pomeranian dog. On the lateral view, the heart is moderately taller than normal. A large bulge is seen at the caudodorsal aspect of the heart representing a severely enlarged left atrium (short arrows). There is dorsal displacement of the trachea, which is almost parallel to the thoracic spine. The left caudal lobar bronchus is also displaced dorsally and compressed by the severely enlarged left atrium (long arrow). On the VD film, the heart is widened and the left cardiac border is rounded and expanded, almost touching the left thoracic wall. Increased soft tissue opacity is seen between the two caudal stem bronchi superimposed on the caudal aspect of the heart almost on midline, representing the enlarged left atrium (short arrows). The lungs are normal with no evidence of left-sided cardiac failure. Diagnosis: moderate cardiomegaly with severe left atrial enlargement. Mitral endocardiosis was found on echocardiography.

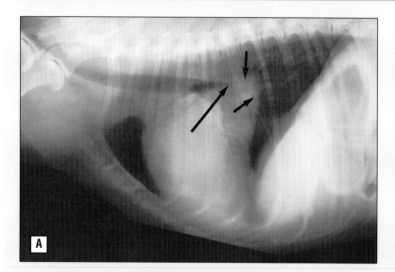
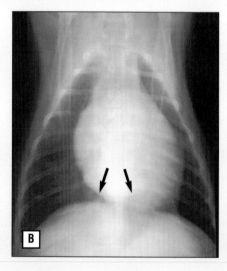

range from normal to severe generalized cardiomegaly (*Figure 5.35*). Cardiogenic edema is common; it can have a rapid onset and is often quite severe. The distribution may be similar to that seen in mitral endocardiosis but often has a diffuse perivascular location or a random, patchy appearance.

HCM is the most common acquired cardiac disease of cats. Radiographic changes include mild to severe left atrial enlargement and mild to moderate right atrial enlargement (*Figure 5.36*). Biatrial enlargement is seen on a VD or DV film as bulges at the right craniolateral (10 o'clock) and left (3 o'clock) borders of the heart and is described as having a "valentine heart" appearance. There is usually no alteration in the size or shape of the left ventricle. Radiographic evidence of failure includes pulmonary venous congestion, which is best appreciated in the hilar zone on the lateral film. Pulmonary edema appears as unstructured interstitial, alveolar, or mixed patterns with a patchy random or perivascular distribution. Pleural effusion is also common.

Infestation by the heartworm *Dirofilaria immitis* occurs in both dogs and cats. Clinically normal or minimally affected animals usually show no appreciable radiographic changes. The mildest abnormalities that may be detected are enlargement of the mid- and peripheral-zone portions of the caudal lobar pulmonary arteries. Larger parasite burdens cause right-sided cardiomegaly, main pulmonary artery enlargement, and enlargement and tortuosity of the pulmonary arteries. Pulmonary infiltrate with eosinophilia is a common allergic response to the worms (*Figure 5.37*). The radiographic features of pulmonary infiltrate with eosinophilia include a moderate to severe unstructured interstitial pattern; moderate to severe bronchial pattern; and, rarely, interstitial nodules. This pattern may make it difficult to see the enlarged pulmonary arteries. Pulmonary infiltrate with eosinophilia may also occur when there is a small parasite load with no cardiac or vascular changes.

Pulmonary thromboembolism is a possible complication to heartworm infestation, especially following adulticide treatment. Although heartworm disease is the most common cause of pulmonary thromboembolism, it also occurs in association with many other diseases that result in hypercoagulable states and cause endothelial damage. The disease has a range of radiographic appearances. Radiographs can be completely normal, which may explain why this disease is diagnosed more frequently postmortem than in the live patient. Radiographic abnormalities include:

❏ Focal or lobar hyperlucency due to absence of blood flow.

❏ Focal or lobar alveolar patterns. Focal alveolar patterns are located at the periphery of the lungs and are wedge

Figure 5.35 Lateral (A) and VD (B) films of a 10-year-old cocker spaniel dog. On the lateral film, there is moderate to severe enlargement of the heart, which measures almost five intercostal spaces wide. The heart is tall and displaces the trachea dorsally. There is also dorsal displacement of the stem bronchi by a large bulge in the area of the left atrium. On the VD film, the heart is widened and rounded. There is indistinct increased opacity of the lungs in the area of the hilus on the lateral film. On the lateral film, there is also mismatch of the cranial lobar vessels with the pulmonary vein (arrows), measuring twice the size of the corresponding artery. Diagnosis: severe cardiomegaly with severe left atrial enlargement, pulmonary venous congestion, and unstructured interstitial pattern in the hilar region of the lung lobes. This most likely represents pulmonary edema. Dilated cardiopathy was found on echocardiography.

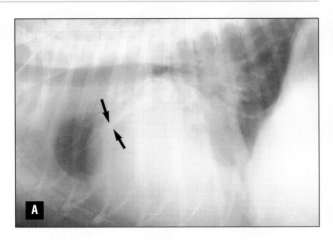

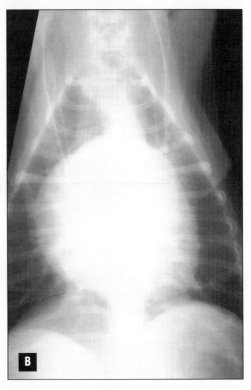

Figure 5.36 Lateral (A) and VD (B) views of the thorax of an adult domestic shorthair cat. The heart is tall, displacing the trachea dorsally on the lateral film. It is also widened, measuring over three intercostal spaces wide. On the VD film, the heart is moderately to severely widened and the cardiac apex is displaced to the right of midline. There is a bulge at the 3 o'clock position of the heart on the VD view, representing enlargement of the left atrial appendage. Patchy increased opacity is present within the lungs, in the hilar and peripheral zones of the caudal lung lobes. This opacity is characterized by an unstructured interstitial pattern that coalesces to form a patchy alveolar pattern. Diagnosis: left-sided cardiomegaly with pulmonary edema. Hypertrophic cardiomyopathy was found on echocardiography.

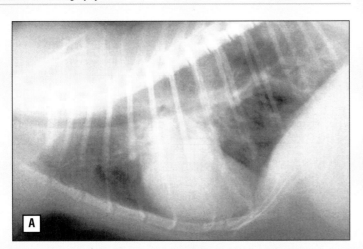

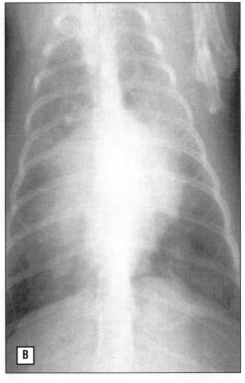

Figure 5.37 Lateral (A) and VD (B) radiographs of the thorax of a 6-year-old domestic shorthair cat. There is moderate to severe enlargement of the right caudal lobar artery, which is seen on the VD radiograph. A moderate, unstructured increase in soft tissue opacity is noted throughout the lung fields. Both heart size and shape are considered to be within normal limits. The arterial abnormality is indicative of heartworm infestation. The unstructured interstitial pattern is consistent with pulmonary infiltrate with eosinophilia. Diagnosis: heartworm disease.

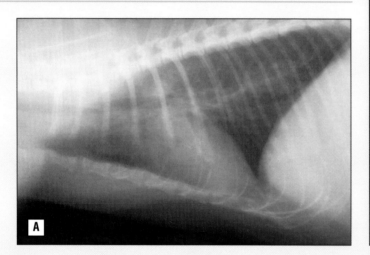

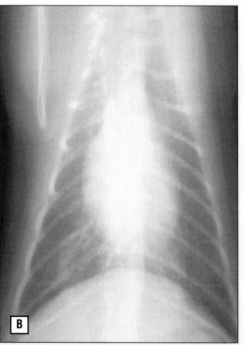

shaped with the apex toward the hilus and the base toward the pleural surface (*Figure 5.38*).

❑ Truncation (abrupt termination) or pruning (absence of normal branches) of the pulmonary arteries and thinning or absence of the pulmonary veins.

❑ Small- or moderate-volume pleural fluid accumulation. If the volume is small, then the fluid may selectively accumulate around the affected lobe.

Definitive diagnosis of pulmonary thromboembolism is difficult and often requires tests, such as selective pulmonary arteriography, pulmonary perfusion scintigraphy, or computed tomography angiography.

Accumulation of fluid within the pericardial sac may occur due to neoplasia, infection, or hemorrhage. In some cases, however, an underlying cause cannot be found. Generalized enlargement of the heart shadow results, with no specific vessel or chamber affected (*Figure 5.39*). The result is often a severe enlargement that has been described as basketball- or pumpkinlike. DCM or atrioventricular valve dysplasia can cause similar severe enlargement. One characteristic feature is a smooth curve forming the caudodorsal border of the heart on the left lateral film.

Pericardial effusion results in right-sided heart failure and pleural fluid accumulation, which may partly or completely obscure the outline of the heart. Congenital peritoneopericardial hernias may mimic pericardial effusion.

Figure 5.38 Lateral thoracic radiograph of a 6-year-old German shepherd dog. The dog had been treated for heartworm disease with an adulticide. There is increased soft tissue opacity in the periphery of the caudal lung lobe. A mottled inhomogeneous opacity partly obliterates the outline of the diaphragm. The increased opacity has a wedge shape, with the base toward the diaphragm and the apex toward the hilus of the lung. Diagnosis: pulmonary thromboembolism.

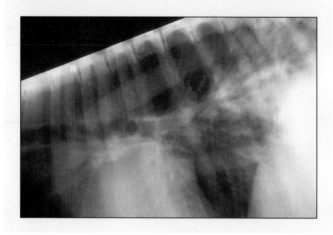

They are often clinically silent and are discovered by accident. A window between the pericardial and peritoneal cavities allows abdominal organs to pass into the pericardium. The heart shadow is severely enlarged, frequently bizarrely shaped, and of inhomogeneous opacity due to the presence of omental and mesenteric fat. Portions of the gas-

Figure 5.39 Lateral (A) and VD (B) radiographs of the thorax of a 7-year-old cocker spaniel dog. The heart is severely enlarged, measuring four and one-half intercostal spaces wide and rounded on the lateral view. Also, the heart is tall causing severe dorsal displacement of the trachea. Similar severe enlargement of the heart silhouette is present in the VD view, with the heart contacting the right thoracic wall and almost contacting the left thoracic wall. No specific cardiac chamber bulges or great vessel enlargements are noted. The lungs are normal. The VD radiograph does not support the increased opacity in the caudal lung lobes on the lateral film. It is most likely an artifact caused by poor inspiratory effort. Diagnosis: pericardial effusion. The presence of a moderate volume of pericardial fluid was confirmed by echocardiography. No evidence of a tumor was found.

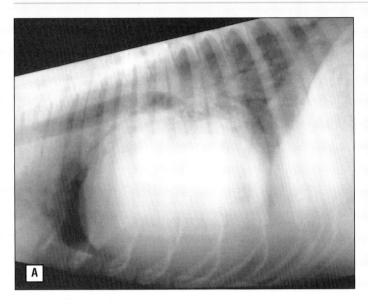
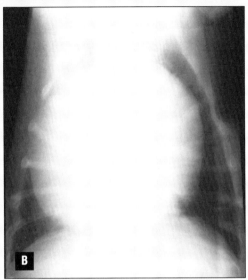

trointestinal tract may be found within the pericardium and, occasionally, animals present with acute-onset intestinal obstruction due to incarceration of the hernia. Echocardiography is required for definitive diagnosis of pericardial disease. Unlike radiographs, which cannot distinguish fluid from the rest of the heart, echocardiography can do so with ease. It can also identify intrapericardial tumors.

The final question in thoracic radiology is whether one has sufficient data to make a confident and safe diagnosis. In many cases the combination of history, clinical findings, and radiologic interpretation yields a diagnosis. If no diagnosis is reached, then the radiologic findings should at least allow decisions to be made about additional tests or immediate treatment.

Alternate Imaging of the Thorax

Although the thorax is well suited to radiographic examination, its complexity also means that other imaging tech-

niques may be needed to obtain a definitive diagnosis. Echocardiography is especially useful in the diagnosis of congenital cardiac disease and assessing the severity of acquired cardiac disease.

Ultrasound can be used to image noncardiac structures. Aerated lung effectively blocks the ultrasound beam; but, if lesions are superficial or there is pleural fluid, a window may be available. Ultrasound can be used to confirm the presence of a mediastinal mass and to evaluate pulmonary masses or consolidations. Perhaps even more helpful, ultrasound provides effective guidance for needle aspirates or biopsies.

Computed tomography is commonly used for thoracic imaging in humans. It is more sensitive than conventional radiography at detecting subtle pulmonary changes, especially small nodules. Because computed tomography is not compromised by air-filled lung as ultrasound is, it offers more accurate guidance when obtaining a biopsy from lesions deep in aerated lung.

Like the thorax, the abdomen is a complex structure and radiographic interpretation is challenging. Unlike the thorax, it is not ideally suited to radiographic examination. Careful attention to technical detail is essential to get the best yield from abdominal radiographs.

Film Quality

The greatest technical problem in abdominal radiology is the relatively small degree of contrast between soft tissue viscera and fat. To maximize the inherent contrast of the abdomen, a low kV(p) and high mA technique should be employed. For abdomens exceeding 10 cm in width or depth, a grid must be used to prevent scatter radiation from fogging the film and further degrading the contrast. The problem of motion blurring can be avoided by making the exposure at the end of expiration when there is usually a brief pause.

Much like the thorax, the large number of structures in the abdomen lends it to a systematic structure-by-structure or organ-by-organ approach to film interpretation. By working through a checklist, one avoids the temptation to focus on an obvious lesion or the organ suspected to be abnormal based on clinical and historical data.

Abdominal Wall and Extra-abdominal Soft Tissues
The Abdominal Wall

Is the wall normal?
Are there any swellings or masses?
Is there evidence of a diaphragmatic hernia?

In a normal cat or dog, the caudal surface of the diaphragm blends with the liver. In animals in fair or better body condition, the inner margin of the abdominal wall is outlined by fat (*Figure 6.1*). Swellings or masses are usually evident clinically and should prompt the observer to evaluate the underlying body wall for evidence of disruption. Diagnosing a diaphragmatic rupture is based on detecting abdominal viscera in the thorax. These organs may be obscured by pleural fluid, and the diagnosis may be difficult.

Secondary changes that suggest a rupture include absence of the normal falciform fat shadow; absence of or cranial displacement of the liver and other viscera; and other signs of trauma, such as rib fractures. Diaphragmatic ruptures can be confirmed by an intraperitoneal injection of a water-soluble iodinated contrast agent at a dose of 400 mg iodine/kg. Any extension beyond the confines of the peritoneal cavity confirms the diagnosis. Alternatively, a small volume of contrast agent may be given orally to confirm the location of the stomach and proximal small intestine.

The Peritoneum and Retroperitoneal Space

What is the patient's body condition?
Is the retroperitoneal space normal?
Is the peritoneal space normal?
Is there retroperitoneal fluid?
Is there retroperitoneal gas?
Is there peritoneal fluid?
Is there peritoneal gas?

Detail within the peritoneal and retroperitoneal spaces is essential for evaluating the abdominal organs. The quality of detail is determined by how much fat is present. This is assessed by looking for subcutaneous fat, retroperitoneal

Figure 6.1 Lateral radiograph of the abdomen of a domestic shorthair cat that had been attacked by a dog. Several loops of small intestine are noted ventral to the abdominal wall. The musculature of the ventral abdominal wall can be traced from the caudal abdomen as a thin soft tissue stripe ventral to the bladder wall. Diagnosis: ventral rupture.

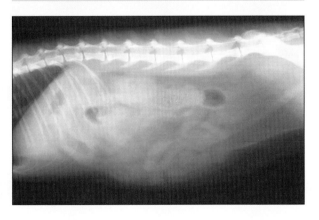

fat, and fat within the falciform ligament ventral to the liver (*Figure 6.2*). When body condition is normal, the complete outline of the left kidney and the caudal pole of the right kidney are visible in the dog. In cats, both kidneys should be clearly outlined. The serosal edges of the abdominal organs and the inner margin of the muscle of the abdominal wall should be clearly visible in an animal in normal body condition (*Figure 6.3*). In animals with no body fat, neither peritoneal nor retroperitoneal organs can be discerned. This is normal in immature patients and is also seen in cachexia due to severe and chronic illness. In cases where

detail is absent due to cachexia, the abdomen has a "tucked-up" appearance.

Retroperitoneal fluid obliterates the outline of the kidneys (*Figure 6.4*). The degree to which the kidneys are obscured depends on the relative quantities of fluid and fat present. When a moderate or large volume of fluid is present, the retroperitoneal space is expanded, causing ventral displacement of the gastrointestinal tract. Possible causes for increased fluid opacity in the retroperitoneum include hemorrhage, urine leakage, neoplasia, and infection. If there is a history of trauma, then the possibility of hemorrhage or urine leakage from a lacerated kidney or a ureter should be considered and can be confirmed or excluded by an excretory urogram. Retroperitoneal gas enhances detail in the dorsal abdomen, and such structures as the abdominal aorta and right kidney are clearly visible. Pneumoretroperitoneum is usually the result of extension of a pneumomediastinum.

Peritoneal fluid accumulation results in a reduction in serosal margin detail, which may be confined to a specific part of the abdomen or generalized. The degree to which detail is lost depends on the relative quantities of fluid and fat present. A small quantity of fluid in a normal or obese animal produces a mottled, wispy, or streaky appearance and blurred serosal edges (*Figure 6.5*). A large volume of

Figure 6.2 Lateral radiograph of the abdomen of a cat. There is complete absence of fat within the peritoneal and retroperitoneal cavities. No subcutaneous fat can be noted. The abdomen has a "tucked-up" appearance. There is complete absence of serosal detail within the abdomen. In this case, there is no abdominal detail because of the complete absence of fat. The shape of the abdomen is the clue that indicates the peritoneal cavity is not filled with fluid. Diagnosis: cachexia. The cat had chronic renal failure.

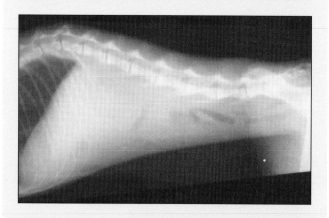

Figure 6.4 Lateral radiograph of the abdomen of a cocker spaniel dog presented collapsed from a gunshot wound. There is increased soft tissue opacity within the dorsal abdomen, obliterating the outline of the kidneys. The gastrointestinal tract is displaced ventrally and compressed by the expanded retroperitoneal space. Serosal detail is still visible in the ventral abdomen indicating this process is confined to the retroperitoneal space. In the caudal thorax, the margins of the lungs are separated from the thoracic wall by soft tissue opacity. A metallic object is noted dorsal to the caudal thoracic spine. Diagnosis: retroperitoneal fluid or mass and pleural fluid. The right ureter had been lacerated by a bullet, causing urine leakage into the retroperitoneal space.

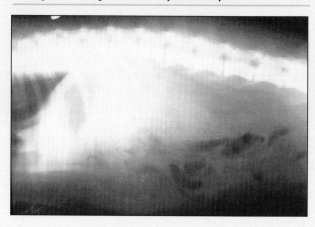

Figure 6.3 Lateral view of the cranial abdomen of a cat. Notice the large amount of fat within the falciform ligament ventral to the liver. A large amount of retroperitoneal fat is also present outlining the kidneys. Note the sharp detail of the serosal borders of the small intestine of the ventral midabdomen. Diagnosis: normal (well-fed) cat.

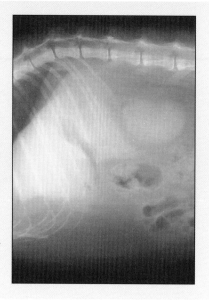

fluid produces a "whiteout" effect, with no serosal detail and usually a few gas-filled loops of intestine floating in the midabdomen (*Figure 6.6*). This may be distinguished from cachexia by the shape of the abdomen and by evaluating retroperitoneal detail and assessing the animal's overall body condition. Many types of fluid can accumulate in the abdomen, including transudates, modified transudates, exudates, blood, urine, chyle, bile, and neoplastic effusions. A small volume of fluid producing a mottled appearance either in part or the entire abdomen is most commonly

caused by peritonitis, hemorrhage, or carcinomatosis.

Peritoneal gas is a grave finding unless abdominal surgery has been performed within the previous 4 weeks. Large or moderate volumes of gas enhance the normal serosal detail (*Figure 6.7*). Normally invisible structures, such as the caudal surface of the diaphragmatic crura and cupola and the caudate lobe of the liver, may be seen. Smaller bubbles are more difficult to detect but can be distinguished by a number of features. These bubbles are evident at the periphery of the abdomen, away from the intestine (*Figure 6.8*). They may

Figure 6.5 Lateral view of the abdomen of a 10-year-old domestic shorthair cat. Note the normal detail within the retroperitoneal space where fat clearly outlines both the kidneys. There is increased soft tissue opacity within the peritoneal cavity, which partly, but not completely, obliterates the serosal margins of the intestines. Diagnosis: moderate volume of peritoneal fluid.

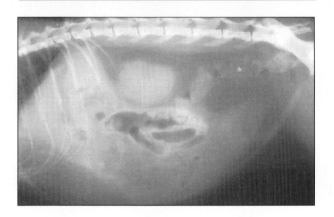

Figure 6.7 Lateral view of the abdomen of a 6-year-old mixed-breed dog. Note that there is a gas bubble in the craniodorsal abdomen, which outlines the caudal surface of the diaphragm and the serosal surface of the fundus of the stomach. A thin curvilinear gas pocket can also be seen between the body of the stomach and the liver in the cranioventral abdomen. Diagnosis: moderate to large volume of free peritoneal gas.

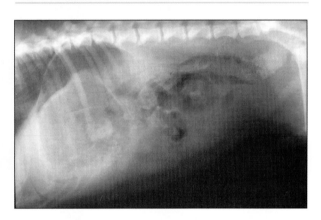

Figure 6.6 Lateral view of the abdomen of a 3-year-old Siamese cat. The abdomen is moderately pendulous. There is no fat within the retroperitoneal or falciform areas. No serosal detail can be seen. There is homogeneous soft tissue opacity within the abdomen. In this cat there is no body fat to supply serosal detail; but the abdomen is distended rather than thin, indicating the presence of fluid. Compare this with *Figure 6.1*. Diagnosis: moderate volume of peritoneal fluid and cachexia. The final diagnosis was feline infectious peritonitis.

Figure 6.8 Close-up view of the cranioventral abdomen of a German shorthaired pointer, which presented collapsed. There is increased soft tissue opacity within the peritoneal cavity, with moderately to severely reduced serosal detail. Multiple, small gas bubbles are seen scattered in the ventral abdomen (arrows). These are not contained within the small or the large intestine. Diagnosis: free peritoneal gas and peritoneal fluid. A perforated duodenal ulcer was also found at surgery.

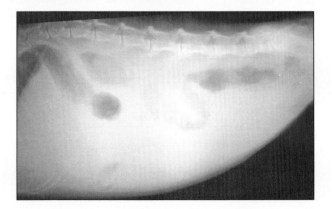

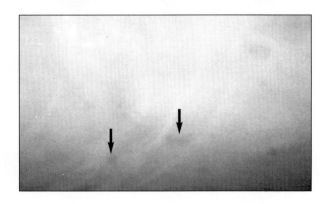

have distinct round shapes, especially if fluid is present, or appear triangular as they outline the serosal edges of adjacent intestinal loops. Free peritoneal air can be confirmed by horizontal-beam radiography. The patient is positioned in left lateral recumbency as that position prevents confusion with the gas bubble in the body of the stomach, and a tightly collimated radiograph is made centered on the right abdominal wall (*Figure 6.9*). Possible causes of peritoneal gas include perforation of the gastrointestinal tract, rupture of an abdominal abscess, or penetrating trauma.

Figure 6.9 VD, horizontal-beam view of the abdomen of a 7-year-old German shepherd cross-breed dog. A large gas pocket is evident beneath the body wall. Note that this radiograph was taken with the dog in right lateral recumbency. The two short arrows indicate the wall of the stomach, the lumen of which contains a small gas bubble. The long arrow indicates the spleen. Horizontal-beam films should be taken with the patient in left recumbency to prevent confusion with the gas pocket in the stomach. Diagnosis: free peritoneal air. At surgery a ruptured liver abscess was found.

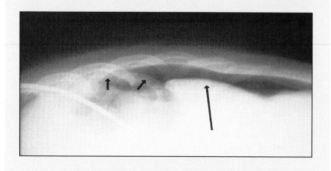

Liver

- Is the liver normal?
- Is the liver too small or enlarged?
- Is the shape of the liver normal?
- Is there gas or mineralization within the liver?

The liver is the largest solid organ in the abdomen. It should have smooth surfaces with lobar edges that form acute angles. Liver size is assessed using the position of adjacent organs and subjective criteria. The normal liver should lie beneath the ribs, extending almost to the arch of the ribs. If one draws a line linking the fundus and pylorus of the stomach, it should lie between perpendicular to the spine and parallel to the ribs on a lateral film in a normal animal. On a VD film, this line should be perpendicular to the spine. A reduction in the size of the liver or cranial displacement of the liver results in cranial tilting of this gastric

axis (*Figure 6.10*). Microhepatia may be caused by congenital portosystemic shunts, chronic hepatitis, or cirrhosis.

Generalized enlargement of the liver causes caudal and dorsal displacement of the stomach and other abdominal viscera (*Figure 6.11*). This finding may be less dramatic in animals with hyperadrenocorticism, as weakness of the abdominal muscles allows the liver to extend ventrally and even severe hepatomegaly may have little effect on the position of the stomach. Extension beyond the ribs may indicate hepatomegaly but should be interpreted carefully as it can be caused by other processes. Any disease that increases the intrathoracic volume displaces the diaphragm and the liver caudally. The liver often extends beyond the ribs in older animals as the ligaments that attach the liver to the diaphragm stretch. Conformational variations may also affect the relative position of the liver and adjacent viscera. Liver size is best assessed based on experience and a subjective assessment of whether the size is appropriate, too large, or too small for the patient.

Intrahepatic lesions may alter the shape of the liver and displace adjacent organs, such as the stomach and right kidney. Blunting or rounding of the normally pointed lobar edges is the best radiographic sign of hepatic disease. Nodules or masses may also protrude from the surface of the liver. One should not mistake for a mass the bulge of a full gallbladder on the ventral surface of the liver in cats.

Intrahepatic mineralization is rare and may be due to mineralized choleliths; parasitic or fungal granulomas; or, rarely, neoplasia. The presence of gas within the liver usually has grave prognostic implications. Linear gas shadows

Figure 6.10 Lateral view of the cranial abdomen of a 1-year-old miniature schnauzer dog. Gas is present within the fundus and body of the stomach. The gastric axis is tilted cranially. The caudoventral margin of the liver does not extend to the edge of the ribs. Diagnosis: microhepatia. A portosystemic shunt was ligated at surgery.

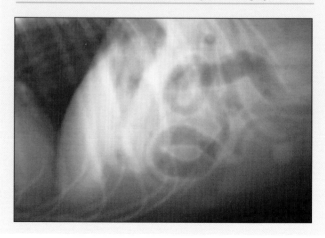

Figure 6.11 Lateral (A) and VD (B) views of the abdomen of an 8-year-old mixed-breed dog. There is caudal and dorsal displacement of the stomach and caudal displacement of the small intestine. The liver extends beyond the ribs, and the caudoventral margin of the liver reaches almost to the level of the umbilicus. On the VD film, there is caudal and leftward displacement of the intestines from the right, cranial, abdominal quadrant. Diagnosis: generalized hepatomegaly. Lymphoma was diagnosed on aspiration biopsy.

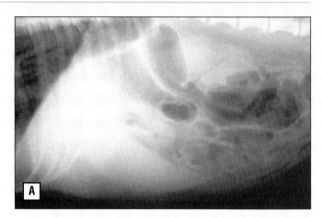

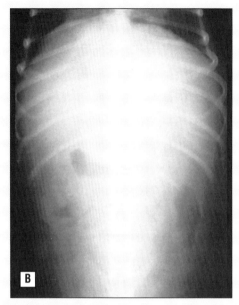

represent gas within the portal veins, hepatic veins, or intrahepatic bile ducts. Intravascular gas may be seen in cases of gastric dilatation-volvulus and indicates mucosal necrosis. A collection of small bubbles may be due to emphysematous cholecystitis (right ventral liver) or abscess formation. Larger bubbles are usually within the gallbladder or an abscess cavity.

Spleen

> Is the spleen normal?
>
> Is there generalized splenomegaly?
>
> Is there a splenic mass?
>
> Is there a splenic torsion?

The spleen is an elongated flat organ with smooth surfaces and borders that form acute angles. The head is held relatively constant in position in the left craniodorsal abdomen by the short gastrosplenic ligament that attaches it to the body and fundus of the stomach. On a lateral film, the head may appear as a flattened, triangular-shaped structure in the craniodorsal abdomen but is not always seen. On a VD film, it appears between the stomach, body wall, and the cranial pole of the left kidney. The body and tail are quite mobile and may be found almost anywhere in the abdomen, depending on the size of the spleen.

In cats, splenic size is quite constant and only the head of the spleen is seen on lateral films. If the tail of the spleen is visible in the ventral abdomen on a lateral film of a cat, then splenomegaly is indicated. Splenic size in dogs

shows considerable variation. Age and activity level have a significant influence. Young, athletic dogs frequently have a "large" spleen; but it is usually small in sedentary or elderly dogs. Such factors as stress also influence splenic size. Phenothiazine tranquilizers and barbiturate anesthetic agents cause splenic congestion and splenomegaly. The best radiographic indicator of pathologic splenic enlargement is rounding or blunting of the edges (*Figure 6.12*).

Figure 6.12 Close-up view of the mid-ventral abdomen of an 11-year-old mixed-breed dog. The spleen is seen lying along the ventral abdominal wall. It extends caudally almost to the bladder. There is slight rounding of the caudal margin of the spleen. Diagnosis: moderate, generalized splenomegaly. Fine-needle aspirates from the spleen were consistent with lymphoid hyperplasia.

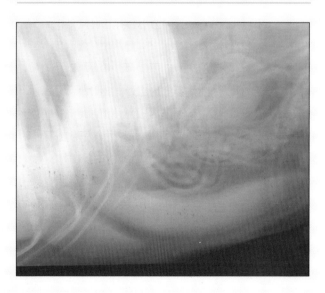

Generalized splenomegaly can be caused by a multitude of processes, including neoplasia, such as lymphoma, venous congestion, hemolysis, extramedullary hematopoiesis, and lymphoid/nodular hyperplasia.

Splenic masses are among the most commonly identified abdominal masses. If located in the body or tail of the spleen, the mass usually lies in ventral midabdomen, causing caudal and dorsal displacement of the small intestine. Tumors, hematomas, abscesses, and cysts may cause masses. The presence of peritoneal fluid may partly or completely obscure a mass, but one should be suspected if there is asymmetric distribution of the small intestine. Splenic torsions may present as large splenic masses accompanied by peritoneal fluid. If there is little or no fluid, then a characteristic, folded, C-shaped spleen may be seen.

Stomach

- **Is the stomach normal?**
- **Is there evidence of pyloric outflow obstruction?**
- **Is there gastric dilation with or without volvulus?**
- **Is there a gastric foreign body?**
- **Is there a gastric wall mass?**

The normal canine stomach lies transversely across the abdomen with the fundus left and dorsal, the body on the left, the pyloric antrum on the right of midline, and the pylorus on the right midway between dorsal and ventral (*Figure 6.13*). In puppies and cats, the stomach has a different anatomic location. On VD film the stomach resembles a J, with the body and fundus on the left and pyloric antrum and pylorus just right of midline (*Figure 6.14*). Obtaining VD, left, and right lateral films, and sometimes a DV film, is recommended in cases of suspected gastric disease. These four different projections move gas and fluid within the lumen and allow evaluation of much of the inner mucosal margin. Stomach and intestinal wall thickness cannot be reliably assessed on survey films because one cannot distinguish gastric wall—either normal or abnormal—from gastric contents of soft tissue opacity. Such an assessment is best done by a contrast procedure or ultrasound.

Chronic partial obstruction of the gastric outflow caused by hyperplasia of the mucosa and muscularis of the pylorus is a disease of small breed dogs. The lesion causes progressively slower gastric emptying and results in gastric dilation. In severe cases, the dilated stomach may extend beyond the umbilicus. The stomach is usually filled with

Figure 6.13 Right lateral (A), VD (B), left lateral (C), and DV (D) views of the cranial abdomen of a dog. Note that gas fills the fundus and body of the stomach on the right lateral projection. On the VD projection, the body and pyloric antrum of the stomach are filled with gas. On the left lateral projection, gas is noted within the pylorus and also distends the descending duodenum. On the DV film, the gas is predominantly located within the fundus. Diagnosis: normal stomach.

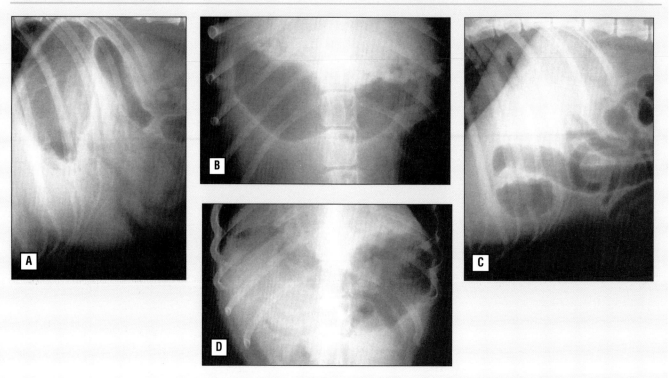

Figure 6.14 VD view of the cranial abdomen and positive gastrogram of a normal cat. Note the shape of the stomach compared with that of a dog (*Figure 6.13*). Puppies' stomachs have a similar appearance to the stomach of this cat. Diagnosis: normal stomach.

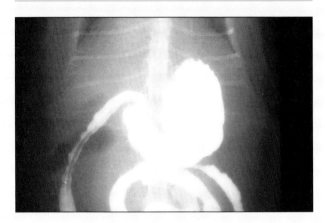

fluid and a smaller quantity of gas. An accumulation of small mineral fragments, the "gravel sign," may be seen in the pyloric antrum due to sedimentation of the heavier, indigestible food particles. The diagnosis may be confirmed

by ultrasound examination. This technique can be used to measure the stomach wall and determine which layers are affected.

Gastric dilatation and volvulus is a life-threatening condition of large and giant breed dogs. If there is severe dilation, then efforts should be directed to relieving that condition before radiographs are obtained. Because animals with gastric dilatation and volvulus are distressed and in shock, the radiographic examination should be quick and minimally stressful. A single, right lateral recumbent film may be sufficient to establish a diagnosis. Alternatively, if the animal will not tolerate lateral recumbency, then a DV film should be made (*Figure 6.15*). One must identify the parts of the stomach and, by deciding if these contain fluid or gas, determine whether they lie left or right of midline. If the stomach is in its normal position, the film will show a gas-filled fundus and body on a right lateral film (*Figure 6.16*). If the stomach has undergone a one-half-turn volvulus, then the pylorus is gas filled and located in the dorsal abdomen, indicating it is left of midline on the upper side of the abdomen. If additional films are required, then a DV and/or left lateral

Figure 6.15 DV (A) and right lateral (B) views of the cranial abdomen of an 8-year-old Gordon setter dog. On the right lateral film, the stomach is moderately distended with gas. The fundus (diamond) is located in the ventral abdomen and is displaced caudally. The pylorus (star) is located in the left cranial abdomen rather than on the right. Diagnosis: gastric dilatation-volvulus.

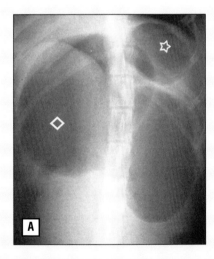

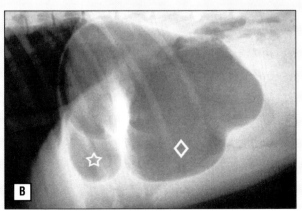

Figure 6.16 DV view of the abdomen of a hound cross-breed dog. Only this radiograph was obtained due to the dog's distressed and painful condition. There is massive gaseous dilation of the stomach. The pylorus (star) is in a normal location in the right cranial abdomen, and the fundus is on the left. Diagnosis: severe gastric dilatation without volvulus.

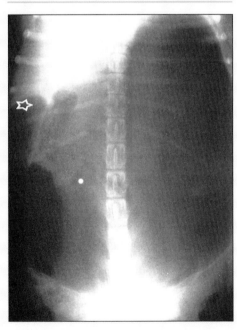

recumbent view may be helpful. It is often easier to identify parts of the stomach if films are obtained after initial decompression. Dilation of the esophagus and generalized severe splenic enlargement are often noted.

The possibility of a gastric foreign body should be considered in animals with unresponsive vomiting and no radiographic evidence of small intestinal obstruction. If a foreign body is suspected, then the radiographic examination consists of a four-view examination of the stomach, that is, left and right lateral, DV, and VD views. A fluid-filled pylorus on the right lateral film can be mistaken for a ball foreign body or mass, as the pylorus often has an almost perfectly round shape and uniform soft tissue opacity. This is an easy trap for the novice radiologist but is readily resolved by taking a left lateral film, which will fill the pylorus with gas.

When a mass is suspected, the animal must be fasted for at least 12 hours, and preferably 24 hours, before radiography. Radiographs are quite insensitive for the detection of gastric masses as most are located along the lesser curvature. The presence of ingesta and fluid within the stomach may mimic wall thickening or obscure a mass. For this reason, neither gastric nor intestinal wall thickness should be assessed from survey radiographs. Suspected gastric tumors are best evaluated by a combination of endoscopy and ultrasound, as the latter technique allows assessment of the liver and regional lymph nodes for metastasis.

Small Intestine

Is the intestine normal?
Is there intestinal dilation?
Is there evidence of a linear foreign body?

The normal small intestine fills the midabdomen and forms multiple, smooth, flowing loops. Normal feline small intestine contains little or no gas and measures no more than 12 mm from serosal surface to serosal surface. Normal canine intestine contains a variable quantity of gas but should not be uniformly gas filled. The serosa-to-serosa width should not exceed 1.6 times the height of the center of the fifth lumbar vertebral body. Intestine should be considered dilated if it exceeds these normal limits. The most common cause of an increased volume of intestinal gas is aerophagia due either to dyspnea or stress, but aerophagia does not cause dilation. When evaluating radiographs, one should be careful not to overlook fluid-filled dilated loops,

which are much less prominent than gas-dilated segments.

Having determined that the small intestine is dilated, one should decide on the severity of the dilation and how much of the intestine is affected. Intestinal obstruction causes dilation of the gut proximal to the lesion. This is usually characterized by moderate to severe dilation of two to three loops proximal to the lesion (*Figure 6.17*). If the obstruction is chronic and distal, then the dilation may extend to involve most of the small intestine. Recent or partial obstructions may demonstrate only limited dilation. Obstruction of the duodenum may also be difficult to confirm, as accumulated secretions are vomited along with gas proximal to the lesion, which prevents the development of dilation. Fabric foreign bodies may act as wicks, allowing the passage of intestinal fluid and minimizing the degree of dilation that develops. Chronic partial obstructions are sometimes accompanied by a gravel sign. In older animals, such obstructions are often due to intestinal tumors. Puppies and kittens may also present a diagnostic dilemma as they have little or no body fat, which hampers identifying dilated, fluid-filled gut. One should be careful to look for the normal gas shadow of the cecum in dogs and the ascending and transverse colon in dogs and cats. Absence of these gas shadows may be a clue to the presence of an ileocolic or cecocolic intussusception.

Figure 6.17 Lateral view of the abdomen of a 2-year-old Labrador retriever dog. There are multiple, moderately dilated segments of small intestine, indicated by the long double-headed arrows. Several of the loops are filled with material that resembles poorly formed feces, and some are distended with gas. The presence of fecal-like material within dilated small intestine is consistent with a subacute to chronic, distal, small intestinal obstructive lesion. The short double-headed arrow indicates the position for measuring the height of L5. All of these small intestinal segments exceed 1.6 times the height of L5. Approximately one third to one half of the small intestine is dilated. Diagnosis: distal small intestinal obstruction.

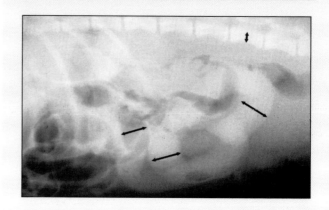

Intestinal dilation may also be caused by paralytic ileus, which commonly produces mild to moderate generalized dilation. Possible causes include spinal injury, abdominal surgery, peritonitis, previous obstruction, polyneuritis, neuromuscular blockade, and pain. Enteritis may also cause generalized dilation. Severe enteritis, such as canine parvovirus infection or hemorrhagic gastroenteritis, may cause moderate to severe dilation of part or all of the gut and may be misdiagnosed as an obstructive pattern. Most patients with gastroenteritis are radiographically normal or have mild generalized dilation.

Linear foreign bodies can be difficult to diagnose. If a foreign body, such as a piece of string, becomes fixed at the base of the tongue, in the pylorus, or in the proximal intestine, the intestine becomes plicated as peristalsis tries to pull the object through. The intestine may have a bunched appearance and look tightly stacked. This tight bunching of the intestine produces abnormal gas bubbles, which appear triangular or comma shaped, unlike the intestine's normal elongated ovoid gas bubbles. These abnormal bubbles are also located eccentrically, that is, toward the edge of the intestinal loops rather than in the center. Linear foreign bodies are a challenging diagnosis and can quickly become life threatening; if a linear foreign body is suspected, then a contrast upper gastrointestinal examination should be performed.

Pancreas

Is the pancreas normal?
Is there evidence of pancreatitis?
Is there a pancreatic mass?

The normal pancreas is small and radiographically invisible. Pancreatitis may produce no radiographic signs, so normal radiographs do not exclude this diagnosis. Moderate to severe pancreatitis triggers a severe inflammatory response in the pancreas and adjacent tissues. This is seen as an ill-defined increased soft tissue opacity within the cranial abdomen along the caudal border of the stomach and the descending duodenum. Caudal displacement of the transverse colon may be seen, with disease affecting the left limb. If the right limb is affected, then there may be lateral and ventral displacement of the descending duodenum. The secondary peritonitis may cause a paralytic ileus of the descending duodenum, which has a fixed, dilated appearance on sequential films. Pancreatic masses cause similar organ displacements. Masses can be due to pancreatitis, pancreatic pseudocysts, or tumors.

Kidneys

Are the kidneys normal?
Are the kidneys small?
Are the kidneys enlarged?
Is the shape normal or irregular?
Is the opacity normal or is there mineralization?

The left kidney is radiographically visible in most dogs in normal body condition; but, in many dogs, only the caudal pole of the right kidney can be seen. Both kidneys should be clearly seen in any cat in normal body condition. Kidney size should be assessed with a VD radiograph as positioning is more constant, minimizing distortion. Normal canine kidneys measure two and one-half to three and one-half times the length of the second lumbar vertebra. Feline kidneys range from two to three times the length of the second lumbar vertebra (*Figure 6.18*). They should have

Figure 6.18 Lateral (A) and VD (B) views of the cranial abdomen of a domestic shorthair cat. Abundant retroperitoneal fat outlines both kidneys. The kidneys are normal in size and shape and have smooth margins and uniform soft tissue opacity. Diagnosis: normal kidneys.

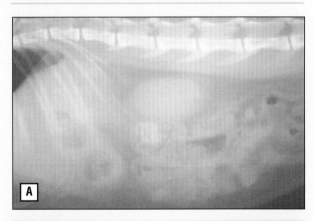

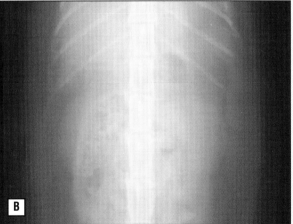

smooth margins and be of homogeneous soft tissue opacity. Canine kidneys are somewhat elongated; feline kidneys are shorter and rounder than canine kidneys.

Small kidneys may be difficult to detect, especially if chronic renal insufficiency leads to cachexia (*Figure 6.19*). In young animals, renal dysplasia or hypoplasia should be considered. In older animals, most forms of chronic acquired renal disease result in a reduction in size; and the kidneys usually have an irregular shape and margin.

Renomegaly may affect one or both kidneys (*Figure 6.20*). Enlargement of the left kidney causes ventral, medial, and caudal displacement of the small intestine and descending colon. Enlargement of the right kidney displaces the descending duodenum and ascending and transverse colon ventrally, medially, and caudally. The small intestine is displaced toward midline, ventrally, and caudally. If the kidney is severely enlarged, then it may be difficult to identify it as the organ of origin. In such cases, the absence of the normal kidney shadow suggests a renal origin of the mass. The shape and margin of the kidney are useful in refining a list of diagnostic differentials. Hydronephrosis, polycystic kidney disease, neoplasia, feline infectious peritonitis, and ethylene glycol poisoning may cause smoothly marginated renomegaly. If the kidney is irregularly marginated, then neoplasia, polycystic kidney disease, and feline infectious peritonitis should be considered.

Urolithiasis is the most common cause of mineral opacity within the kidney (*Figure 6.21*). Uroliths may conform to the shape of the pelvis and diverticula and have a staghorn shape. Some uroliths are soft tissue rather than mineral opacity (**c**ysteine and **u**rate, "I can't **C U**") and can only be detected by a contrast study or ultrasound. Small, focal, parenchymal mineralizations are common in chronic renal disease.

Figure 6.19 VD view of the cranial abdomen of a cat. The right kidney is small and slightly irregularly shaped. A small irregularly shaped mineral opaque structure is seen in the area of the renal pelvis. The left kidney is at the lower end of the normal range and slightly irregularly shaped. Diagnosis: chronic renal disease.

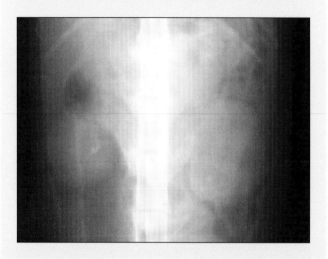

Figure 6.20 Lateral view of the abdomen of a cat. The small and large intestine are displaced ventrally and caudally by two homogenous, well-defined ovoid soft tissue masses in the dorsal midabdomen (arrows). Normal kidney shadows cannot be seen. Diagnosis: severe, bilateral renomegaly. Renal lymphoma was diagnosed by fine-needle aspirate.

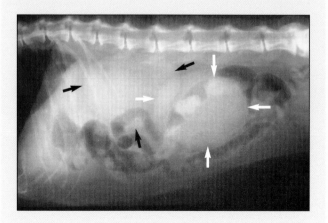

Figure 6.21 Lateral abdomen of a terrier cross-breed dog. Multiple, irregularly shaped, mineral opaque uroliths can be seen within the lumen of the urinary bladder. Note that there are multiple uroliths also within the penile urethra caudal to the os penis (arrow). In cases of suspected urolithiasis in male dogs, a film centered on the penile urethra, with the animal's legs pulled forward, should always be obtained. Diagnosis: urocystolithiasis and urethral obstruction by uroliths.

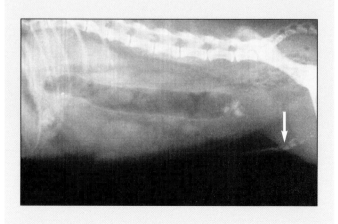

Bladder

Is the bladder normal?

Is the bladder enlarged?

Is the shape normal or irregular?

Is the opacity normal or is there mineralization?

Is the bladder intact?

The bladder lies in the caudoventral abdomen. A normal canine bladder is pear shaped with the neck located just cranial to the pubis; feline bladders are more round than and located more cranial to the pubis than canine bladders. Normal bladder size is difficult to define; but, if the bladder extends cranial to the umbilicus, diseases that cause urine retention should be considered. Tumors seldom alter the shape or opacity of the bladder. In rare cases, the contour of the bladder neck may be distorted or there may be nebulous, poorly defined mineralization within the tumor.

If a tumor is suspected, then one should remember to search for enlarged sublumbar lymph nodes. Suspected bladder tumors should be investigated by contrast radiography and ultrasound because they seldom produce survey radiographic abnormalities. Uroliths may range from an accumulation of sandlike material to large stones. When uroliths are detected or suspected in male dogs, an additional film of the penile urethra must be obtained. Cysteine and urate uroliths are soft tissue opacity and cannot be detected on survey radiographs. They require contrast radiography or ultrasound for diagnosis.

Bladder rupture may occur as a result of blunt abdominal trauma or urethral obstruction. Rupture usually releases a moderate to large volume of fluid into the peritoneal cavity with a consequent reduction in peritoneal detail. The absence of a normal bladder outline with the presence of peritoneal fluid warrants a positive contrast cystogram to confirm or exclude a rupture.

Prostate

Is the prostate normal?

Is the prostate enlarged?

Is the shape normal or irregular?

Is there evidence of a prostatic carcinoma?

The normal prostate is contained within the pelvis. It may lie within the abdomen in young dogs, when pulled cranially by a full bladder, and in normal older dogs. In a large breed dog, the prostate is approximately the size of a walnut. Enlargement causes cranial displacement of the prostate and the bladder and dorsal displacement and compression of the colon (*Figure 6.22*). If severe, constipation may result and the colon is filled with very opaque, well-formed fecal material. Benign prostatic hyperplasia, prostatitis, abscessation, cysts, paraprostatic cysts, and carcinomas cause prostatic enlargement. If the gland is asymmetrically enlarged, then abscessation, cyst formation, or neoplasia is more likely.

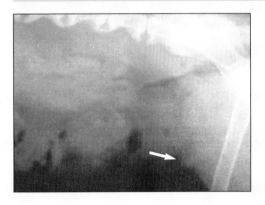

Figure 6.22 Lateral view of the caudal abdomen of a boxer dog. There is cranial displacement of the bladder by a mildly to moderately enlarged, rounded prostate. The prostate has homogenous soft tissue opacity and has smooth margins. Note the normal triangular fat opacity between the caudoventral aspect of the bladder, cranioventral aspect of the prostate, and abdominal wall (arrow). There is no evidence of enlargement of the sublumbar lymph nodes. Diagnosis: moderate prostatomegaly. The final diagnosis was benign prostatic hyperplasia.

Prostatic carcinomas are variable in size. Radiographically detectable sublumbar lymph node enlargement supports a diagnosis of neoplasia. Irregularly marginated, palisadelike new bone on the ventral cortex of the last two to three lumbar vertebrae, sacrum, and first few caudal vertebrae indicates tumor invasion of these structures.

Uterus and Ovaries

Is the uterus normal?

Is the uterus enlarged?

Is there evidence of a pregnancy?

Are there signs of fetal death?

Is there a cause for dystocia?

Is there an ovarian mass?

The normal uterus and ovaries are radiographically invisible, although the body of the uterus may sometimes be seen between the bladder neck and colon in obese animals. Enlargement of both uterine horns produces a characteristic displacement of the small intestine toward midline and dorsally and cranially (*Figure 6.23*). Pregnancy cannot be distinguished from pathologic causes of uteromegaly until fetal mineralization has occurred after day 42 (*Figure 6.24*). After day 50 of pregnancy, the fetal skeletons can be used to count the number of puppies or kittens in a litter.

Fetal death is more readily detected by ultrasound, as radiographic changes take up to 24 hours to develop. The fetus may adopt a hyperextended or hyperflexed posture. There may be collapse and overlap of the skull bones; and, if putrefaction has begun, intrafetal and intrauterine gas may be present. In cases of dystocia, radiographs can diagnose fetal malposition or fetopelvic mismatch.

Ovarian masses tend to gravitate to the ventral midabdomen and cause displacement of the small intestine toward midline and away from the affected side. Ovarian tumors often contain mineralization.

Figure 6.23 VD view of the abdomen. There are homogeneous soft tissue structures in the left and right caudal abdomen. These structures have displaced the small intestine cranially and toward midline. This is a characteristic pattern of displacement caused by uterine enlargement. Diagnosis: moderate uteromegaly. Pyometra was diagnosed by ultrasound.

Figure 6.24 Lateral view of the midabdomen of a dog. A soft tissue structure present in the mid-ventral abdomen causes cranial and dorsal displacement of the small intestine. Within the soft tissue structures, multiple, fetal, mineral skeletal structures can be seen. Diagnosis: pregnancy.

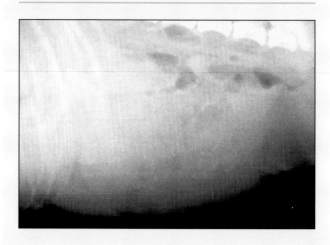

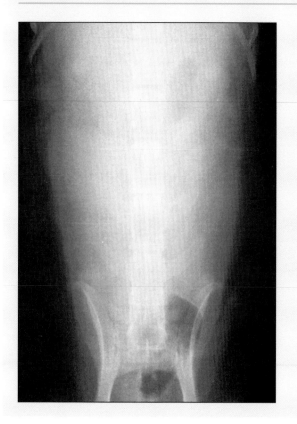

In essence, ultrasound is used to image tissues much as sonar is used to find fish or submarines and radar is used to find aircraft. A short pulse of energy, which for ultrasound is high frequency sound, is produced in the transducer by a crystal that converts electrical energy to sound. The sound pulse is sent into the tissue. The same transducer then listens for an echo or echoes produced when the sound pulse is reflected from structures within the tissue, and these echoes are converted back into very weak electrical signals. A computer processes the echoes, and the data are used to construct the image. The sound used is generally in the range of 2 to 10 MHz, much higher in frequency than the human ear's normal audible range of 50 Hz to 20 kHz, hence the term *ultrasound*.

The image is constructed by assuming that sound travels at a constant speed in all tissues, so the time taken for the echo to return is directly related to the distance traveled. Thus the time for the sound pulse to travel out into the tissue and back to the transducer is used to determine the depth of the object and where it is displayed on the monitor. The intensity of the returning echo determines the brightness of the object on the screen. An image is constructed from thousands of echoes, each of which produces a point of varying intensity at a specific position on the screen, making a two-dimensional representation of the patient being examined. Two-dimensional, real-time ultrasonography is sometimes referred to as B-mode, or brightness mode. B-mode imaging is the modality routinely used for abdominal ultrasound and for echocardiography.

The Routine Abdominal Ultrasound Scan

Ultrasonographic examination of the abdominal organs is much like reading radiographs in that one must be systematic and thorough to avoid overlooking lesions. To become a competent ultrasonographer, it is essential to develop a pattern of scanning that one follows all the time. The approach does not matter, so long as all of the organs are scanned completely. An examination is performed much like reviewing an abdominal radiograph, by scanning each organ in turn for normalcy or evidence of disease.

One approach is to begin at the liver, applying the probe at the ventral midline just caudal to the xyphoid process. The liver is scanned by angling the probe back and forth to left

and right and then rolling the probe 90° to obtain transverse images. The spleen is next, scanned by sliding the probe dorsally along the left ribs all the way to the head of the spleen. Usually to ensure seeing all of the spleen requires three to four scans from tail to head. The left kidney is imaged next, and then the stomach is scanned from left to right, followed by scanning the right kidney. The midabdomen is scanned in a crisscross pattern until the bladder and prostate or uterus are reached. Having completed the basic scan, one should return to evaluate small organs, such as the adrenal glands, pancreas, uterus, ovaries, and lymph nodes. An alternative method is to scan in clockwise direction, beginning at the liver, then spleen, left kidney, stomach, small intestine on the left, uterus, bladder, prostate, and small intestine on the right and right kidney.

Liver

> **Is the liver normal?**
> **Are there focal parenchymal abnormalities?**
> **Is the hepatic parenchyma diffusely hyperechoic, hypoechoic, or mottled?**
> **Is the biliary system normal?**
> **Are the portal and hepatic veins normal?**

When evaluating the liver one should assess the parenchyma, the biliary system and the vasculature. Normal hepatic parenchyma has a finely granular texture; and the echogenicity is equal to (isoechoic), or slightly greater (hyperechoic) than, the cortex of the right kidney and less than (hypoechoic) the spleen. The surface of the liver is smooth and the lobar borders form sharp points. Portal vein branches within the liver can be distinguished from hepatic veins by their hyperechoic walls, due to the presence of fat and fibrous tissue (*Figure 7.1*). The walls of the hepatic veins blend with the liver parenchyma, and the veins become larger as they converge on the caudal vena cava. The gallbladder is round and tapers toward the neck (caudally) and is quite variable in size. It may seem quite large in anorexic or fasted animals, and that does not usually indicate biliary obstruction. Its wall blends with the liver parenchyma and is smooth. Normal bile is anechoic; but echogenic sludge is common, especially in fasted or anorexic patients (*Figure 7.2*).

Figure 7.1 Transverse view of the liver of a normal dog. Note the liver parenchyma has a granular, slightly coarse, uniform echotexture. Two large blood vessels cross the field of view. The deeper vessel with the hyperechoic wall is a portal vein. The more superficial vessel is a hepatic vein. Normal hepatic arteries and biliary ducts are not visible. Diagnosis: normal liver.

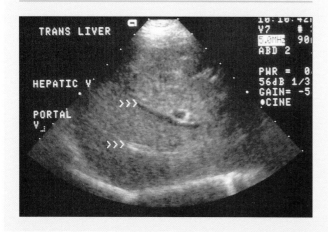

Figure 7.3 Sagittal scan of the liver of a terrier dog. An irregularly marginated, bilobate, hyperechoic mass is noted within the liver parenchyma. Diagnosis: hyperechoic liver mass. On additional images, several similar masses were noted. The histologic diagnosis after biopsy was nodular hyperplasia.

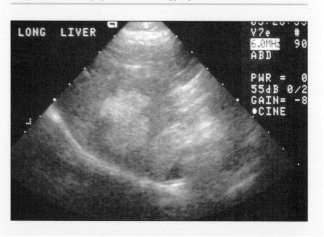

Figure 7.2 Transverse view of the liver of a normal dog. The ovoid, dark structure on the left of the image is a normal gallbladder. Note that the gallbladder contents are anechoic. Diagnosis: normal liver.

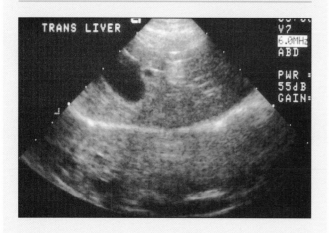

Focal hepatic abnormalities include masses, nodules, and cysts. Such lesions may be hypoechoic or hyperechoic in comparison to normal liver parenchyma or mixed echogenic. The differential diagnosis for focal lesions includes cysts, abscesses, primary or metastatic neoplasia, hematomas, granulomas, extramedullary hematopoiesis, and nodular hyperplasia (Figure 7.3). Ultrasonographic characteristics of focal and diffuse lesions are quite nonspecific, and ultrasound-guided biopsy/aspiration is always required for a definitive diagnosis.

Detection of diffuse hepatic parenchymal abnormalities is based on comparison of the echogenicity of the parenchyma to adjacent reference organs and structures.

The relative visibility of the portal markings should also be assessed. Diffuse disease may cause the liver to be hyperechoic, hypoechoic, mottled, or normal. Liver size and shape are best assessed on radiographs, but the margins of the liver can be assessed by ultrasound and a "guesstimate" can be made regarding liver size.

A diffusely hyperechoic liver is isoechoic to the spleen and more echogenic than the kidney cortex and portal veins are difficult to see. This may be caused by steroid hepatopathy (iatrogenic, Cushing's disease), lipidosis, diabetes mellitus, fibrosis, chronic active hepatitis, neoplasia, and cirrhosis (*Figure 7.4*). A diffusely hypoechoic liver is less echogenic than the spleen and kidney cortex, and the portal veins are very prominent (sometimes called the "starry night effect"). This may be caused by acute hepatitis, cholangiohepatitis, neoplasia, congestion, and hepatic necrosis. A diffusely mottled liver may have an overall increase or reduction in echogenicity. Possible causes include hepatic necrosis, toxins, diffuse abscessation, hepatitis, fibrosis, and cirrhosis. Hepatic lymphosarcoma most commonly appears normal but may be diffusely hyperechoic, diffusely hypoechoic, or have multiple hypoechoic nodules or masses.

Choleliths are occasionally found in companion animals but rarely cause clinical problems. Inspissated bile, referred to as mucoceles or sludgeballs, appear similar to sludge but do not change shape in response to movement. These may be associated with cholecystitis, seen as thickening of the gallbladder wall or biliary obstruction. Dilation of the com-

Figure 7.4 Sagittal image of the liver of a 15-year-old domestic shorthair cat. There is uniform increased echogenicity within the liver. The arrows outline the capsule of the liver; and, superficial to that location, there is falciform fat. Normally the falciform fat is more echogenic than the liver. The portal veins cannot be seen due to the increased parenchymal echogenicity. Diagnosis: uniformly hyperechoic liver. The cytologic diagnosis was hepatic lipidosis.

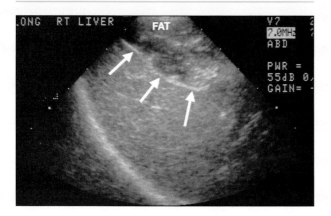

Figure 7.5 Dorsal plane image in the left cranial abdomen of a normal dog. The spleen is visible in the near field. A single splenic vein can be seen within the splenic parenchyma and penetrating the capsule of the spleen at the hilus. The bright hyperechoic line to the right and below the spleen is gas and fecal material within the colon. Diagnosis: normal spleen.

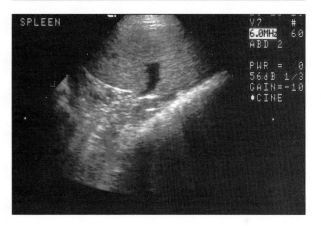

mon bile duct may be seen with both obstruction and cholangiohepatitis. Ultrasound is relatively insensitive in detecting biliary obstruction.

Hepatic venous distension may be found in cases of right-sided heart failure or partial obstruction of the caudal vena cava, such as in heartworm disease. The extrahepatic and intrahepatic portions of the portal veins can also be evaluated to detect portosystemic shunts.

Spleen

Is the spleen normal?

Are there focal parenchymal abnormalities?

Is the splenic parenchyma diffusely abnormal?

Are the splenic veins normal?

Location of the body and tail of the spleen is variable. The tail can lie in the right ventral abdomen caudoventral to the gastric body or extend as far caudal as the bladder. Because of the variable location, the spleen is best examined by first locating the head and then sliding the transducer probe along the spleen's length. The normal canine splenic parenchyma has a fine echotexture and is hyperechoic to both the liver and left renal cortex (*Figure 7.5*). The head of the spleen may fold on itself resulting in the appearance of "two spleens," in the left dorsal abdomen. Multiple splenic veins along the hilus penetrate the visceral splenic surface.

The splenic capsule appears as a hyperechoic border when the ultrasound beam is perpendicular to the capsule.

Focal splenic lesions include primary and metastatic neoplasia, hematomas, nodular or lymphoid hyperplasia, extramedullary hematopoiesis, abscesses, infarcts, and cysts. Focal lesions may be solitary or multiple (*Figure 7.6*). Many splenic nodules are benign, and hyperechoic splenic nodules are almost always caused by benign processes (such as nodular hyperplasia or fibrosis). Hematomas are common causes of splenic masses and must be distinguished from hemangiosarcoma (HSA). The gross and ultrasonographic appearances of these two splenic lesions are identical; and, thus, the two processes cannot be distinguished except by histology. Both appear as complex mixed echoic masses, which frequently contain fluid-filled cavities.

With lymphosarcoma (LSA), splenic lesions are more common than hepatic lesions. LSA in the spleen may cause single or multiple hypoechoic to anechoic nodules or masses. Many diffuse splenic diseases may cause generalized splenomegaly, which can be difficult to assess by ultrasound, but frequently do not alter the appearance of the parenchyma. LSA may also cause a diffuse alteration in echogenicity with a honeycomb or "Swiss cheese" appearance (*Figure 7.7*). A similar appearance may be seen in some cases of splenic torsion. Thrombosis of the splenic veins is most common with torsion but may occur as an isolated event.

Figure 7.6 Sagittal image of the tail of the spleen in a poodle dog. A solitary, well-defined, hypoechoic nodule is seen within the parenchyma of the spleen. Diagnosis: splenic nodule. The cytologic diagnosis was extramedullary hematopoiesis.

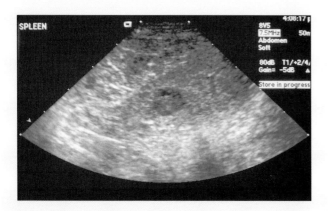

Figure 7.7 Sagittal image of the spleen of a Persian cat. The splenic parenchyma is mottled with multiple, small, hypoechoic nodules. The remaining splenic parenchyma is identical in appearance. Diagnosis: multiple nodules. The cytologic diagnosis was lymphoma.

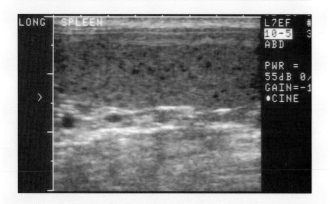

Kidney

Is the kidney normal?

Are there cysts, masses, or nodules?

Are there uroliths or parenchymal mineralization?

Is the parenchymal echogenicity increased?

Is there dilation of the renal pelvis?

The right kidney in dogs is more difficult to image because it is located relatively cranial under the ribs. It can be imaged either using a lateral approach through the last two or three intercostal spaces or from the ventral abdomen medial to or caudal to the last rib. The canine left kidney is imaged through the left ventral or lateral abdominal wall,

just caudal to the ribs. Feline kidneys are located more caudally, with both lying caudal to the ribs. The fibrous tissue of the renal pelvis and peripelvic fat in the renal hilus are hyperechoic. The normal pelvic lumen and ureter are not seen. The cortex is hyperechoic to the medulla, which is quite dark and almost anechoic (*Figures 7.8 and 7.9*). The echogenicity of the cortex of the right kidney is hypoechoic or isoechoic to the caudate lobe of the liver, and the left kidney is hypoechoic to the spleen. The cortices of normal feline kidneys appear much more echogenic because of fat deposition within tubular cells.

Renal cysts are round and well defined, with anechoic or slightly echoic contents and distal acoustic enhancement. Small cortical cysts are common with chronic renal disease.

Figure 7.8 Sagittal image of the left kidney of a normal dog. Note that the medulla is dark, almost anechoic. The cortex is uniformly echogenic with a fine granular echotexture. Diagnosis: normal kidney.

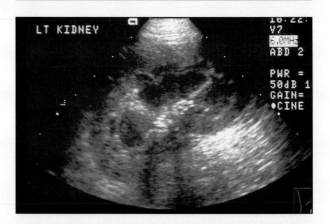

Figure 7.9 Sagittal plane image of the left kidney of a cat. The medulla is almost anechoic, and there is sharp distinction between the medulla and cortex. The cortex is more echogenic than is normally seen in a dog. This is due to fat deposition within tubular cells, which is normal in cats. Diagnosis: normal kidney.

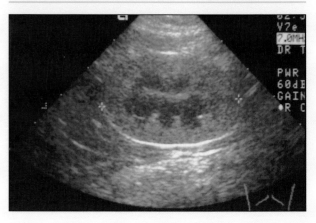

Polycystic kidney disease is a heritable disease in Persian and Himalayan cats, and multiple cysts are usually present by 1 year of age (*Figure 7.10*). Renal nodules and masses are usually neoplastic and may have a mixed echoic, hypoechoic, or hyperechoic appearance. Renal LSA in cats can cause renomegaly, usually with normal internal renal architecture, hypoechoic cortical nodules, and mild pyelectasia. There may be a band of hypoechoic tissue between the cortex and capsule, resulting in generalized enlargement. This may also be seen with granulomatous feline infectious peritonitis.

Figure 7.10 Sagittal image of the kidney of a 3-year-old Persian cat. No normal renal architecture is seen. Multiple, thin-walled, cystic structures that contain anechoic or mildly echogenic fluid are notable. Diagnosis: polycystic kidney disease. The sonographic appearance of the right kidney was similar.

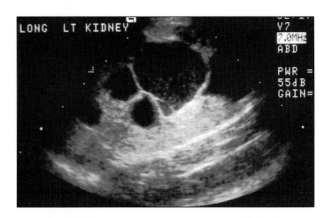

Renal calculi appear as discrete hyperechoic foci in the pelvis and diverticula. They reflect the ultrasound beam because their mineral content causes an acoustic shadow, a dark streak that results from absence of any ultrasound transmission. Small calculi may not be large enough to cause an acoustic shadow. Small parenchymal foci of mineralization may be seen with many chronic renal diseases.

It is nearly impossible to distinguish among the many types of chronic acquired renal diseases based on the ultrasound appearance alone. Normal or enlarged kidneys with normoechoic or hyperechoic cortices, good cortico-medullary distinction, and normal shape may be seen with diseases causing acute renal failure. Small, irregularly shaped, kidneys with increased medullary and cortical echogenicity causing poor corticomedullary distinction are seen with most chronic diseases and renal dysplasia. Almost all of the chronic acquired renal diseases cause an increase in cortical and medullary echogenicity. Definitive diagnosis requires biopsy but usually has little effect on treatment or prognosis.

A few renal diseases have relatively specific ultrasound appearances. Ethylene glycol poisoning rapidly produces an intense increase in cortical echogenicity (*Figure 7.11*). Ultrasound can be used to confirm suspected poisoning within just a few hours of ingestion. Hypercalcemia has been reported to produce a hyperechoic band at the junction of the cortex and medulla of the kidney, although this appearance also occurs in dogs and cats with no evidence of renal disease. A hyperechoic medullary band adjacent to the pelvis has been described with canine leptospirosis. Other nonspecific abnormalities include increased cortical echogenicity, perinephric effusion, and pyelectasia.

Diuresis or pyelonephritis can cause mild pelvic dilation or pyelectasia. Ureteral obstruction is more likely to cause moderate to severe hydronephrosis.

Figure 7.11 Sagittal plane image of the left kidney of a 2-year-old German shepherd dog. There is an intense increase in echogenicity within the renal cortex. Also there is less dramatic increase in echogenicity within the medulla. The kidney is outlined by a moderate to large volume of anechoic fluid. Diagnosis: increased renal and medullary echogenicity. This was a case of ethylene glycol intoxication.

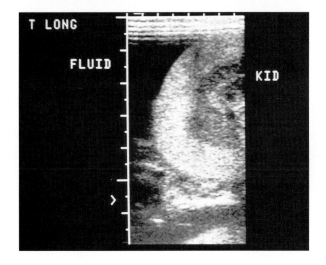

Gastrointestinal Tract

Are the stomach and the small and large intestine normal?

Is the wall thickness increased and are the wall layers disrupted?

Is there a mass of gastrointestinal origin?

Is the small intestine dilated or obstructed?

The stomach, descending duodenum, and colon lie in relatively fixed anatomic locations and are easily identified. The jejunum is coiled randomly in the midabdomen. The wall of the stomach and small intestine has five alternating hyperechoic and hypoechoic bands corresponding to the mucosa, submucosa, muscularis, and serosa and the mucosa-lumen interface (*Figure 7.12*). Normal wall thickness for the canine stomach is 3 to 5 mm and for small intestine is 2 to 3 mm.

An increase in wall thickness with or without disruption of the five sonographic layers may occur with inflammatory bowel disease or infiltrative neoplasia. Thickening that produces obliteration of the normal layers is more commonly seen with tumors. GI masses associated with lymphoma are relatively easy to diagnose in cats, as the species usually has little gas in the intestine. Masses or infiltrative lesions can be obscured by gas, especially in the stomach, however, so ultrasound should be considered an insensitive test.

Figure 7.12 Sagittal (A) and transverse (B) images of normal small intestine of a dog. Note the alternating hyper- and hypoechoic bands within the wall of the intestine, which is best seen on the sagittal image. In the transverse image, the intestine resembles a coffee bean. Diagnosis: normal intestine.

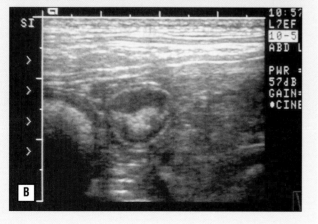

Figure 7.13 Transverse plane image from the ventral midabdomen of a dog. Two moderately dilated, fluid-filled segments of small intestine are evident. In real-time imaging, there was no evidence of peristalsis. Several other similar loops were noted. There were also several loops of normal small intestine. Diagnosis: regional, moderate, small intestinal dilation. An intestinal obstruction was confirmed surgically.

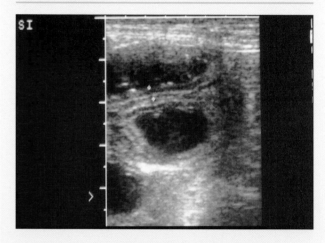

Intestinal obstruction can be difficult to diagnose ultrasonographically but may be suspected if the bowel is dilated (*Figure 7.13*). This may only be detected if the bowel is filled with fluid rather than gas. Obstructions can be easily overlooked if a moderate or large volume of gas is present. The ultrasonographic features of small intestinal obstruction are the presence of dilated, fluid-filled loops proximal to the obstruction and normal loops distal to it. The bowel may be hypermotile if the obstruction is recent or hypomotile if more chronic. An intussusception has a characteristic appearance of multiple concentric layers with a segment of gut and hyperechoic fat in the center.

Bladder

Is the bladder normal?
Are there uroliths?
Is there evidence of cystitis?
Is there a mass lesion of the bladder wall?

Normal urine is anechoic and the normal bladder has a smooth, well-defined wall. A full bladder is ovoid and tapers towards the neck. A nearly empty or partly filled bladder may have an irregular shape as it is indented by the adjacent colon and small intestine. The normal feline bladder is more spheroid with a blunt rather than a tapered neck. Transducer pressure can compress the bladder shape and excessive pressure may collapse or displace a partly filled bladder.

Ultrasonography can be used with greater sensitivity than radiographs to detect uroliths. Calculi appear as intraluminal hyperechoic structures with distal acoustic shadowing (*Figure 7.14*). Urolithiasis is commonly accompanied by cystitis. Cystitis usually causes thickening of the wall at the apex of the bladder but can cause diffuse bladder wall thickening in severe or chronic cases (*Figure 7.15*). In chronic cystitis the mucosa may appear irregular and the mucosal interface may be hyperechoic. Polyps may project into the lumen from affected portions of the wall, usually at the apex.

Figure 7.14 Sagittal image of the bladder of a 6-year-old bichon frisé. Three hyperechoic structures are seen in the dependent portion of the urinary bladder. Dark streaks are visible deep in these hyperechoic structures, representing acoustic shadowing. Diagnosis: urocystolithiasis.

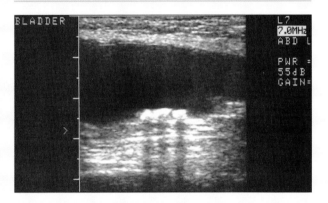

Figure 7.15 Sagittal image of the bladder of a 5-year-old Maine coon cat. There is moderate thickening of the urinary bladder wall, which measures 3 to 4 mm thick. A moderate amount of sediment is seen in the dependent portion of the urinary bladder (arrow). There is an indistinct outpouching from the bladder lumen at the apex of the bladder (long arrow). Diagnosis: chronic severe cystitis with suspicion of a urinary bladder diverticulum, such as a urachal remnant. This was confirmed at surgery.

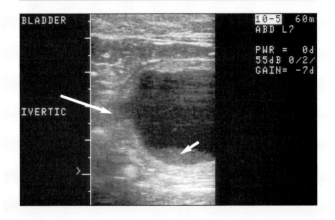

Transitional cell carcinoma is the most common neoplasm of the urinary bladder. These tumors generally appear as mixed echoic or hyperechoic cauliflowerlike masses projecting into the lumen. Tumors occur most commonly in the bladder neck and trigone (*Figure 7.16*). Intraluminal blood clots are hyperechoic or mixed echoic and may have a complex echotexture and irregular, ill-defined margins. They can be misdiagnosed as a mural mass, especially when they are adhered to the bladder wall; but, unlike masses, clots may move when the bladder is balloted and change in appearance as the clot matures. The regional lymph nodes adjacent to the aorta and the iliac arteries should always be evaluated in cases of suspected neoplasia of the bladder. Fine-needle aspirates from the lymph nodes may be more helpful than urine sediment cytology in obtaining a diagnosis.

Figure 7.16 Sagittal plane image of the neck of the bladder of a 10-year-old beagle dog. A mass of homogeneous echogenicity is indicated, outlined by long arrows. This appears to originate from the ventral wall of the neck of the bladder. The arrowhead indicates the vesicourethral junction. The mass has a homogeneous echogenicity with hyperechoic mucosal border. Diagnosis: bladder neck mass. A transitional cell carcinoma was diagnosed on aspiration biopsy.

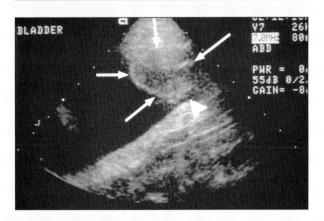

Normal Uterus and Ovaries

> **Are the uterus and ovaries normal?**
> **Is there evidence of pyometra?**
> **Is there evidence of pregnancy?**
> **Is there evidence of fetal death?**

The normal uterus is best located by imaging in a transverse plane in the caudal half of the bladder. The cervix and uterine body are seen as a round structure dorsal to the bladder and ventral to the colon. The uterine horns are smaller in diameter than the body and are usually not seen if normal. Normal ovaries are difficult to identify and are located adjacent to the caudal poles of the kidneys.

Pyometra causes the uterine horns to enlarge and fill with pus, which varies from anechoic to hyperechoic (*Figure 7.17*). The disorder may sometimes cause asymmetric or focal uterine enlargement. Hydrometra and mucometra also cause uterine enlargement but are less common.

Ultrasonography has several advantages over radiography in pregnancy detection. It can be used to confirm pregnancy much earlier than radiographs, in the beginning of the second trimester. Fetal viability can be verified by

detecting a heartbeat and fetal movement (*Figure 7.18*). The major disadvantage of ultrasonography is that the technique provides only a rough estimate of litter size. Pregnancy diagnosis is most reliably performed between day 25 and day 30 of pregnancy. At that point, the fetus can be seen as a small ovoid structure within a sac filled with anechoic fluid, and the fetal heartbeat is visible. Lack of a fetal heartbeat and absence of fetal movement indicate fetal death. These signs are seen several hours before radiographic changes indicative of fetal death develop.

The Prostate and Testes

> Is the prostate normal?
> Is the prostate enlarged?
> Are there parenchymal abnormalities?
> Are there cavities within the prostate?

The normal prostate gland is often located in the pelvic canal and may be difficult or impossible to image. In older dogs a normal prostate is more likely to be within the abdomen, especially if pulled cranially by a full bladder. A normal prostate is hypoechoic to the surrounding tissues, appearing slightly fusiform in the longitudinal section and round and bilobed in the cross section (*Figure 7.19*).

Benign prostatic hyperplasia is the most common prostatic disease. It causes symmetrical enlargement with uniformly hyperechoic parenchyma. If the parenchyma has a

Figure 7.17 Transverse scan of the uterus of an 8-year-old greyhound dog. The uterus is moderately enlarged and the uterine horns are distended with mildly echoic to anechoic fluid. Diagnosis: pyometra.

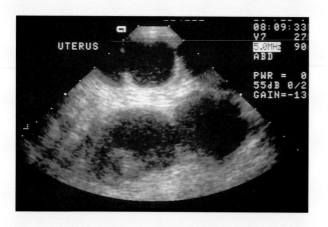

Figure 7.18 Ultrasound image of a canine fetus at approximately day 30 of gestation. This is a sagittal plane fetal image. The small, rectangular, hyperechoic structures represent the vertebrae. The heart can be seen surrounded by lungs. In real-time imaging, the heartbeat was detected. The liver can also be identified in this image. Diagnosis: normal pregnancy.

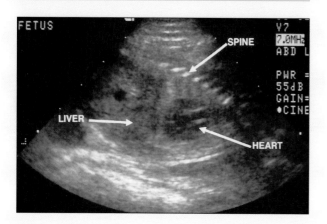

Figure 7.19 Transverse image of the prostate of a recently neutered 2-year-old springer spaniel dog. The prostate is small, measuring approximately 1.5 cm in width, and has a slightly inhomogeneous hypoechoic echogenicity. The capsule is smooth and even. Diagnosis: normal prostate.

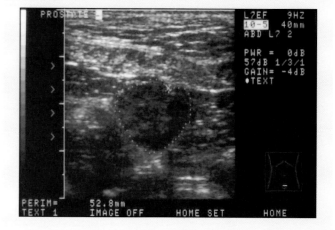

mixed or mottled echogenicity, bacterial infection and neoplasia should be considered. Bacterial prostatitis usually has mixed echoic parenchyma (*Figure 7.20*). A severe infection may extend to involve adjacent peritoneal fat, which will appear hyperechoic; and sometimes a small volume of adjacent peritoneal fluid is noted. Prostatic neoplasia does not have any characteristic features. Abscessation and carcinoma may occur in the same patient.

Figure 7.20 Sagittal image of the prostate of a 7-year-old terrier cross-breed dog. The prostate is enlarged, measuring 3 cm in depth. The parenchyma has a mottled, hypoechoic appearance. Diagnosis: prostatomegaly with abnormal parenchyma. Prostatitis was diagnosed by aspiration biopsy.

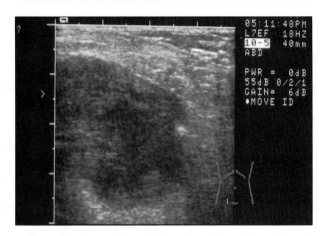

Mineralization may occur with chronic inflammatory disease and carcinoma but is more often associated with prostatic tumors. The sublumbar lymph nodes should always be examined when prostatic abnormalities are seen. The lymph nodes enlarge with both inflammatory and neoplastic prostatic disease. If the lymph nodes are sufficiently large, then they should be aspirated.

Multiple cysts with anechoic contents may be seen within the prostate in cases of benign hyperplasia. Cavitated lesions with echogenic contents are suggestive of abscess formation but abscess contents vary in echogenicity from anechoic to almost isoechoic with the parenchyma. An abscess that is sufficiently large can cause asymmetric enlargement. Cavitated lesions may also be seen with carcinomas.

Testes

Are the testes normal?
Are there parenchymal abnormalities?

Normal testicular parenchyma has a uniform parenchyma, comparable in echogenicity to the spleen and has finely granular echotexture. The mediastinum testis is identified as a thin, linear, hyperechoic structure in the center of the testicle (*Figure 7.21*). Neoplastic testicular masses can be solitary but are more often multiple and present in both testes. Almost all tumors, regardless of type, appear as hypoechoic nodules.

Figure 7.21 Sagittal image of the testicle of a 10-year-old German shepherd dog. A solitary, well-defined, hypoechoic nodule is present within the parenchyma of the caudal pole of the testicle. Note the hyperechoic structure at the center of the testicle, which is the mediastinum testis. Diagnosis: testicular tumor.

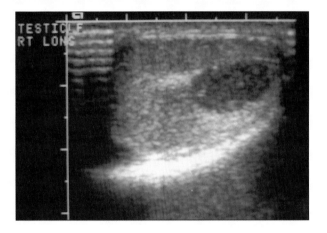

Adrenal Glands

Are the adrenal glands normal?
Is there adrenal gland enlargement?
Is there an adrenal mass?

The adrenal glands are easiest to locate using vascular landmarks rather than the kidneys. The left adrenal gland is ventrolateral to the aorta, cranial to the left renal artery, and at the level of or immediately caudal to the origin of the cranial mesenteric artery (*Figure 7.22*). The right adrenal gland is dorsal or dorsolateral to the caudal vena cava, at the level of or immediately cranial to the cranial mesenteric artery (*Figure 7.23*). Normal canine adrenal glands

Figure 7.22 Scan of the left dorsal midabdomen of an 8-year-old dachshund dog. The aorta (AO) is seen as a dark stripe that stretches obliquely across the image. The arrows indicate the left renal artery. Cranial to the artery and lateral to the wall of the aorta, the adrenal gland is seen as a well-defined, peanut-shaped, hypoechoic structure. The size of the adrenal gland is within normal limits. Diagnosis: normal left adrenal.

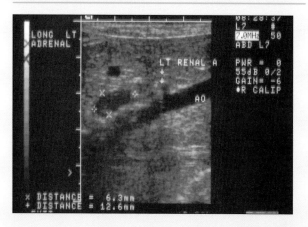

Figure 7.23 Scan of the right cranial abdomen of a beagle dog. In the near field, the caudal vena cava is compressed by transducer pressure. The well-defined, hypoechoic, peanut-shaped structure dorsal to the caudal vena cava is the right adrenal gland. The size and echogenicity are within normal limits. Diagnosis: normal right adrenal gland. Note the close relationship to the caudal vena cava.

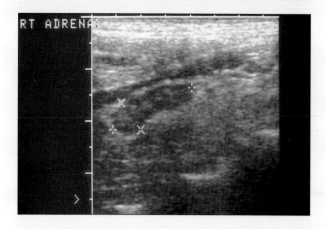

are hypoechoic to the surrounding fat and should measure less than 7 to 8 mm in depth at their caudal poles.

Pituitary-dependent hyperadrenocorticism (PDH) accounts for 80% to 85% of dogs with hyperadrenocorticism. In dogs with PDH, the adrenal glands may appear ultrasonographically normal or symmetrically enlarged (often described as "plump"). A diagnosis of PDH cannot be made without appropriate abnormal adrenal function test results.

Adrenal masses may be caused by primary or metastatic neoplasia and hyperplasia. Most adrenocortical tumors are nonfunctional and are serendipitous findings during an ultrasound examination performed for some other reason. They may appear as focal nodular enlargement of the adrenal or a mass. Adrenal-tumor hyperadrenocorticism (ATH) caused by functional adrenocortical tumors accounts for 10% to 20% of dogs with naturally occurring hyperadrenocorticism. Pheochromocytomas may arise from the medulla and may not be suspected because there are no clinical signs or clinical signs that are nonspecific. The ultrasonographic appearance of pheochromocytomas is similar to that of other adrenal tumors. It is relatively common to find nodules in the adrenal glands on a routine abdominal examination. These nodules present a diagnostic dilemma when there is no clinical evidence of adrenal disease. Noninvasive tests of adrenal function and serial ultrasound monitoring are recommended.

Dogs with malignant tumors may be presented for clinical signs related to invasion of surrounding tissues, especially the caudal vena cava or lumbar spine. Adenomas and carcinomas have similar appearances ultrasonographically, appearing as a mixed echoic, hyperechoic, or isoechoic mass (*Figure 7.24*). Calcification is found in both adenomas and carcinomas. Invasion by the mass of adjacent vessels or tissues indicates that the tumor is a carcinoma and is one of the few features that can be used to distinguish malignant from benign adrenal tumors.

Figure 7.24 Dorsal plane image of the right abdomen of a dachshund dog. A well-defined, mixed, echogenic mass is seen at the lateral aspect of the caudal vena cava (CVC). The mass was in the area of the right adrenal gland, and a normal right adrenal gland could not be identified. Diagnosis: right adrenal gland mass.

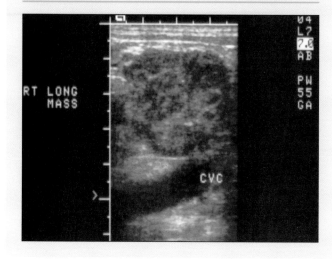

Pancreas

Is the pancreas normal?

Is there pancreatitis?

Is there a pancreatic mass?

The normal canine pancreas is difficult to evaluate with ultrasound because the gland's small, thin shape makes it hard to identify, because it is very similar in echogenicity to surrounding fat, and because of gas within the adjacent GI tract. The pancreas is divided into three parts: right limb, left limb, and head. The right limb lies in the mesoduodenum dorsomedial to the descending duodenum and ventral to the right kidney and caudate lobe of the liver. The pancreaticoduodenal vein lies in the right limb and courses parallel to the descending duodenum (*Figure 7.25*). The head of the pancreas lies caudodorsal to the pylorus and craniomedial to the right kidney. The left limb lies caudal to the stomach, extending across the midline almost to the left kidney and the spleen.

Canine pancreatitis has a range of ultrasonographic appearances depending on the severity and duration of the disease process. In severe pancreatitis, extensive steatitis and peritonitis caused by pancreatitis appears as amorphous, hyperechoic tissue, which the ultrasound beam may not penetrate, thus obscuring the diseased pancreas. If the pancreas can be seen, it is a hypoechoic structure surrounded by hyperechoic, peripancreatic fat (*Figure 7.26*).

Figure 7.25 Sagittal plane image of the right cranial quadrant of a 6-year-old mixed-breed dog. In the near field, there is a segment of descending duodenum. Between the two cursors deep to the duodenum, there is a portion of the right limb of the pancreas. The pancreaticoduodenal vein is seen as two, parallel, hyperechoic lines in the center of that portion of the pancreas. Diagnosis: normal pancreas.

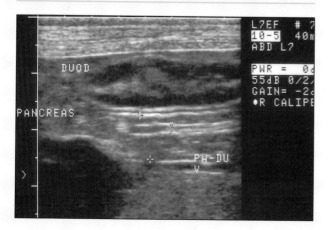

Figure 7.26 Sagittal plane image of the right cranial quadrant of a 5-year-old terrier cross-breed dog. The descending duodenum is in the near field. Deep to the descending duodenum, there is an irregularly marginated, hypoechoic structure. This is surrounded by intensely hyperechoic fat. The hypoechoic structure represents a moderately to severely enlarged pancreas. The hyperechoic tissue is reactive and inflamed fat. Diagnosis: moderate to severe pancreatitis.

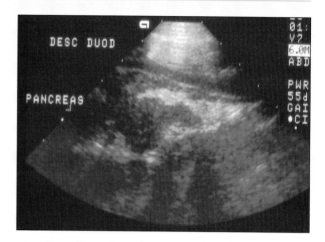

Peripancreatic fluid, duodenal paralytic ileus, and biliary tract obstruction may be seen with severe pancreatitis. Some dogs with pancreatitis show no ultrasonographic abnormalities.

Pancreatic neoplasia is uncommon compared with pancreatitis. Pancreatic adenocarcinomas are highly malignant, and regional metastasis to the liver and lymph nodes has often occurred by the time of presentation. Pancreatic adenocarcinomas frequently resemble cases of acute pancreatitis and may only be distinguished by cytologic or histologic examination. Insulinomas are rare, are usually small, and are extremely difficult to detect. The presence of enlarged regional nodes or hepatic metastases may be helpful changes.

Abdominal Lymph Nodes

Are the lymph nodes normal?

Is there lymph node enlargement?

Normal abdominal lymph nodes may be invisible ultrasonographically because their echogenicity is similar to that of fat. All normal lymph nodes are elongated, thin, fusiform structures. The medial iliac lymph nodes are located lateral to the caudal vena cava or aorta between the deep circumflex iliac and external iliac vessels. Lymph nodes are also located adjacent to the portal vein at the hilus of the liver, around the splenic veins, at the root of the mesentery, and along the mesenteric border of the intestine.

Lymph nodes become hypoechoic and enlarged and, thus, ultrasonographically visible as a result of inflammation, metastasis, or lymphosarcoma (*Figure 7.27*). Such changes may reflect either a specific disease in a structure drained by the node or a generalized/multicentric process, such as lymphosarcoma. Detection of enlarged lymph nodes should prompt the examiner to evaluate carefully the organs drained by the nodes.

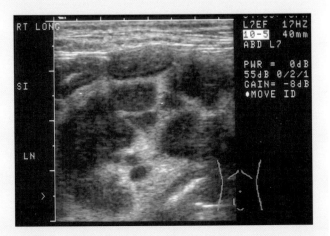

Figure 7.27 Sagittal plane image of the midabdomen of a cat. Multiple, well-defined, ovoid, hypoechoic structures are evident, surrounded by small intestine. These have uniform echogenicity. Diagnosis: moderately to severely enlarged mesenteric lymph nodes. Lymphoma was diagnosed by aspiration biopsy.

CASE 1

SIGNALMENT: 8-year-old mixed-breed dog
REASON FOR PRESENTATION: left forelimb
    lameness

Figure 8.1 Craniocaudal view of the distal antebrachium and carpus of the dog. A mixed productive and destructive lesion is seen within the distal diaphysis and metaphysis of the radius. There is moth-eaten lysis of the radius. Irregularly marginated, well-mineralized new bone can be seen along the medial cortex of the distal radius. The location and appearance of this lesion are consistent with a primary malignant bone tumor. There is, however, also a destructive lesion within the proximal portion of the fifth metacarpal bone and complete lysis of the affected portion of the metacarpal. The presence of two lesions is atypical for a primary malignant bone tumor and suggests metastatic neoplasia or disseminated osteomyelitis. A bone scan was performed to evaluate the skeleton.

Figure 8.2 Lateral skeletal scintigraphy images of the dog's right and left forelimbs and the thorax. There is intense focal tracer accumulation in the distal left antebrachium (1) and proximal left metacarpus (2). A focal area of increased uptake is also noted in the area of the olecranon of the left ulna (3). The focal radiotracer accumulation in the midportion of the right antebrachium (4) represents contamination from the intravenous injection of the radioactive tracer. A mild to moderate focal increased uptake can also be identified in the right eighth rib. Further, focal increased uptake is present in two sites in the cranial thoracic spine.

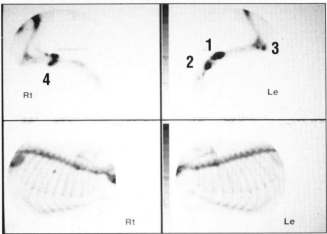

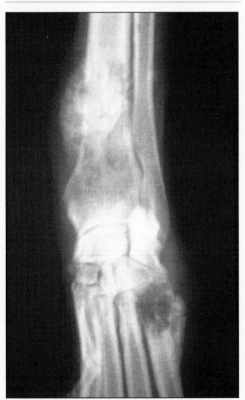

Figure 8.3 Lateral view of the left elbow. A moth-eaten lytic lesion is noted within the olecranon. This has an ill-defined border and no evidence of new bone production. The appearance is similar to the fifth metacarpal lesion shown in *Figure 8.1*.

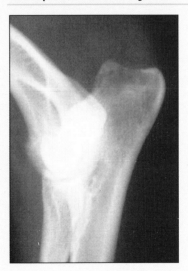

Figure 8.4 Close-up view of the right side of the thorax. Smoothly marginated new bone formation is notable on the medial aspect of the right eighth rib. No evidence of bone lysis is visible.

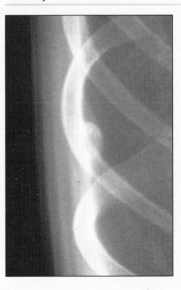

Diagnosis: polyostotic, aggressive skeletal lesions

Case comments: The appearance of the distal radial, fifth metacarpal, and ulnar lesions is consistent with metastatic skeletal neoplasia or, less likely, fungal osteomyelitis. The rib lesion does not appear as active or aggressive but probably represents the same disease process. Repeating the radiographs in 2 to 4 weeks to assess for progression of the lesion would be helpful. A metastatic carcinoma was diagnosed by biopsy.

CASE 2
SIGNALMENT: 2-year-old Doberman pinscher dog
REASON FOR PRESENTATION: repair of distal radial and ulnar fractures

Figure 8.5 Craniocaudal (A) and lateral (B) views of the distal antebrachium of the dog. These radiographs were obtained immediately after surgical repair of oblique fractures of the radius and ulna. A bone plate and multiple screws have been used to stabilize the fracture. The alignment and reduction of the fracture are satisfactory.

Figure 8.6 Lateral (A) and craniocaudal (B) views of the distal antebrachium of the dog. The second set of radiographs was obtained 6 weeks after the initial repair. There is moderate to severe soft tissue swelling surrounding the distal antebrachium. Abundant, irregularly marginated, poorly to moderately well-mineralized new bone is noted on the distal radius and ulna extending some distance from the fractures.

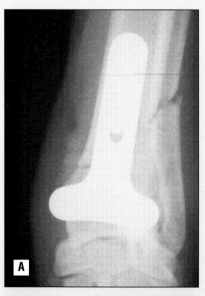

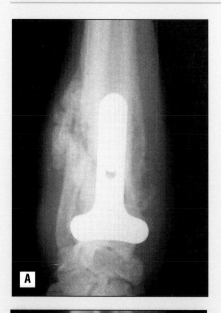

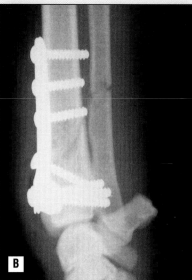

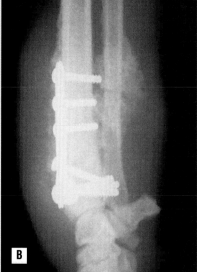

Diagnosis: osteomyelitis

Case comments: Internal fixation with a plate and screws is relatively rigid and should heal with minimal formation of callus. In this case there is exuberant aggressive new bone formation. This could be the result of instability, but there is no evidence of implant failure or loosening. The soft tissue swelling also points to osteomyelitis as the diagnosis.

CASE 3

SIGNALMENT: 11-year-old flat-coated retriever dog
REASON FOR PRESENTATION: history of bloody nasal discharge for 2 months and recent painful swelling over right frontal sinus

Figure 8.7 Rostrocaudal view of the frontal sinus (A), ventrodorsal open-mouth view of the nasal chambers (B), and oblique view of the right frontal sinus (C). There is increased soft tissue opacity within the right frontal sinus and ill-defined loss of bone at the lateral aspect of the sinus. The oblique view demonstrates a large defect in the frontal bone, which has irregular moth-eaten margins. There is soft tissue swelling superficial to this defect. The ventrodorsal open-mouth view (B) demonstrates increased soft tissue opacity within the right caudal nasal chamber with destruction of the nasal and ethmoid turbinates.

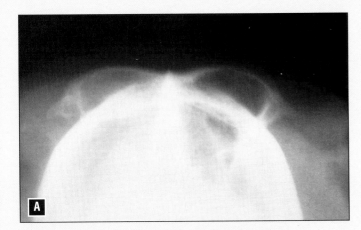

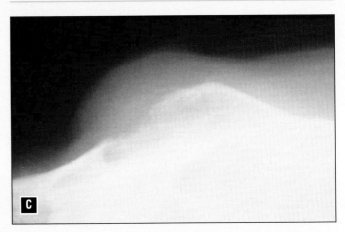

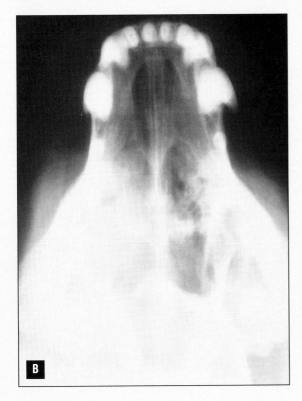

Figure 8.8 A magnetic resonance scan was performed for treatment planning. In this sagittal plane image, the tumor mass is indicated by the star. The arrows indicate extension of the tumor mass into the calvarium.

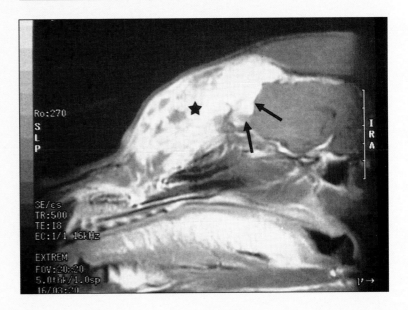

Diagnosis: nasal and frontal sinus neoplasia with invasion of the calvarium

Case comments: The moth-eaten destruction of the frontal bone indicates this is a very aggressive lesion. Malignant neoplasia is the most likely diagnosis.

CASE 4

SIGNALMENT: 11-year-old dachshund dog
REASON FOR PRESENTATION: history of gradual
   onset exercise intolerance

Figure 8.9 Lateral (A) and ventrodorsal (B) views of the thorax. There is a homogeneous increased soft tissue opacity in the cranial thorax, which obliterates the outline of the heart. The trachea is displaced dorsally and to the right. On the ventrodorsal view, this soft tissue mass is seen to be on midline. It displaces the left and right cranial lung lobes caudally and laterally.

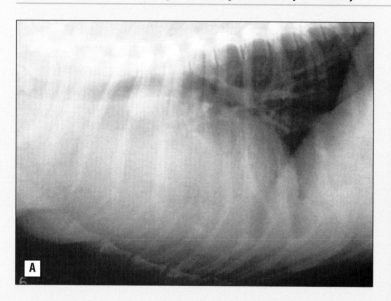
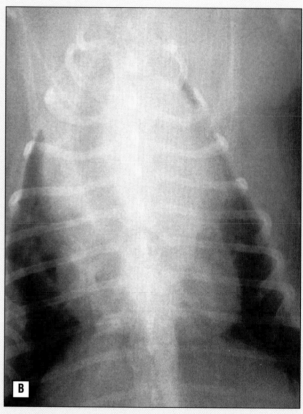

Diagnosis: cranial mediastinal mass

Case comments: The differential diagnosis for this mass includes mediastinal lymph node or thymic lymphoma, thymoma, ectopic thyroid carcinoma, or heart-base tumor. The histologic diagnosis was chemodectoma.

CASE 5

SIGNALMENT: 3-year-old mixed-breed dog
REASON FOR PRESENTATION: hit by car
    immediately before being presented; tachypneic
    and agitated on physical examination; fractured
    right femur

Figure 8.10 Ventrodorsal (A) and lateral (B) radiographs of the dog's thorax. In the ventrodorsal view, there is increased soft tissue opacity in the left caudal hemithorax, which obliterates the outline of the heart and the left side of the diaphragm. On the lateral film, there is increased soft tissue opacity in the caudal thorax, which obliterates a portion of the outline of the cupola of the diaphragm and the caudal cardiac border. The two arrowheads indicate the diaphragmatic crura. A gas-filled structure is noted in the caudodorsal thorax (longer arrows). This represents the fundus of the stomach, which lies cranial to the diaphragmatic crura.

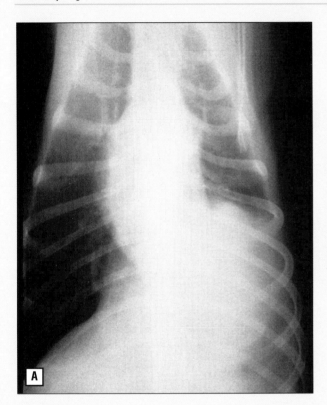

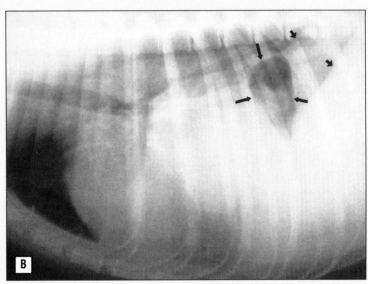

Diagnosis: diaphragmatic rupture with herniation of the liver and a portion of the stomach in the thorax

Case comments: Detecting a part of the gastrointestinal tract within the thorax makes the diagnosis of a hernia straightforward. Doubt about whether the stomach and intestine are in their normal positions can be resolved by giving a small volume of contrast agent orally to confirm the position of the proximal gastrointestinal tract. An alternative is to inject water-soluble iodinated contrast medium into the peritoneal cavity and look for leakage into the pleural cavity.

CASE 6

SIGNALMENT: 4-year-old mixed-breed dog
REASON FOR PRESENTATION: recently acquired
    from the animal shelter; presenting complaint of
    coughing and exercise intolerance

Figure 8.11 Lateral (A) and ventrodorsal (B) films of the thorax. The cranial cardiac border is rounded and the heart is widened on the lateral radiograph. The right cardiac border is rounded on the ventrodorsal view, and the heart has a reversed-D type appearance. A large bulge is seen at the 1 o'clock position on the heart—the location of the main pulmonary artery—on the ventrodorsal view. There is moderate to severe enlargement of the left and right caudal lobar arteries (arrows). There is a moderate increase in unstructured pulmonary opacity. This is most severe at the periphery of the lung fields on the lateral film.

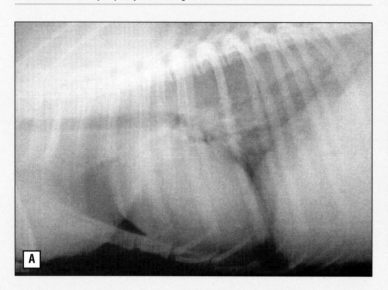

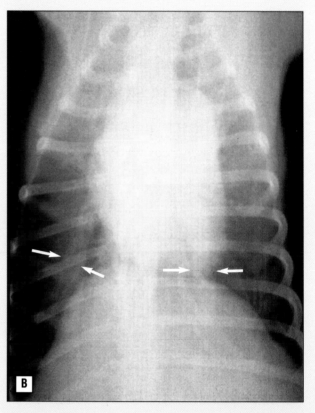

Diagnosis: heartworm disease and pulmonary infiltrate with eosinophilia

Case comments: The cardiac and arterial changes in this dog indicate a moderate to large parasite burden. The unstructured interstitial pattern is a common presentation of pulmonary infiltrate with eosinophilia. Remember, this may occur without any cardiac or vascular changes.

CASE 7

SIGNALMENT: 6-year-old Irish setter dog
REASON FOR PRESENTATION: acute onset of vomiting, which did not respond to conservative management; muffled heart sounds noted on physical examination. Dog has always had intermittent gastrointestinal upsets.

Figure 8.12 Lateral (A) and ventrodorsal (B) views of the thorax. There is severe enlargement of the heart silhouette, which causes dorsal displacement of the trachea. On the ventrodorsal view, the heart contacts both thoracic walls. There are multiple tubular gas-filled structures at the caudoventral aspect of the heart silhouette on the lateral film. These are loops of small intestine, some of which are mildly to moderately dilated. In the ventrodorsal view, there is cranial displacement of the body of the stomach in the left cranial abdomen. The cupola of the diaphragm blends with the outline of the heart.

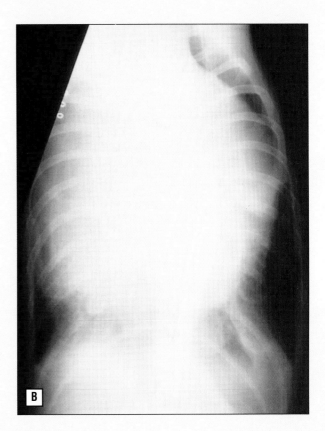

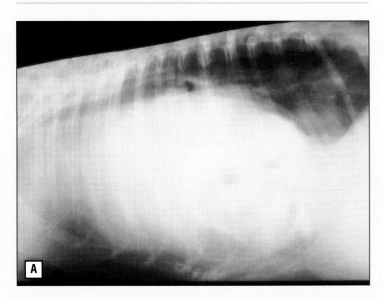

Diagnosis: peritoneopericardial hernia with displacement and incarceration of the small intestine causing obstruction

Case comments: Peritoneopericardial hernias are congenital anomalies and are frequently clinically silent. Occasionally, as in this dog, displacement of part of the intestine results in obstruction or strangulation and the acute onset of clinical signs.

CASE 8

SIGNALMENT: 9-year-old domestic shorthair cat
REASON FOR PRESENTATION: severe dyspnea;
history of chronic hacking cough

Figure 8.13 Lateral (A) and dorsoventral (B) views of the thorax. In the lateral view, the diaphragm is pushed caudally and flattened. In the ventrodorsal view, the thorax is wide causing a barrel-chested appearance. There are multiple doughnut-type markings within the lung fields, which indicates the presence of a bronchial pattern. The lung fields are markedly overinflated.

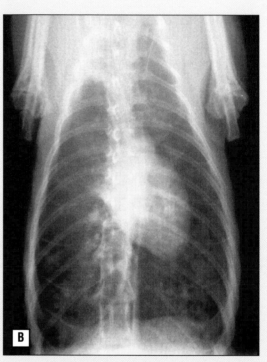

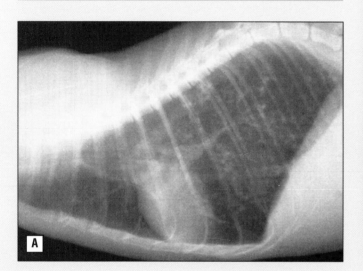

Diagnosis: feline asthma

Case comments: There is severe air trapping resulting in overinflation of the lung fields. This cat has a moderate bronchial pattern, but the appearance of the lung changes is ameliorated by the overexpansion and causes one to underestimate the severity of the pattern. If the lungs contained a normal volume of air, then the pattern would be denser and appear more severe.

CASE 9

SIGNALMENT: 2-year-old Labrador retriever dog
REASON FOR PRESENTATION: acute-onset
vomiting with no response to treatment

Figure 8.14 Left (A) and right (B) lateral radiographs of the cranial abdomen of the dog. The right lateral radiograph is normal. On the left lateral radiograph, a homogeneous soft tissue opacity structure is noted within the lumen of the stomach (arrows). Note the normal gas-filled pylorus in this view (★).

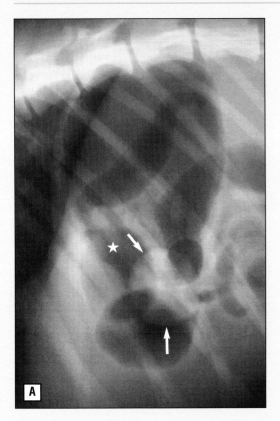
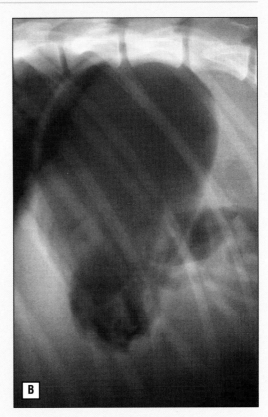

Diagnosis: gastric foreign body

Case comments: A ball was recovered at surgery. The canine pylorus often fills with fluid on right lateral projections and appears as a perfectly round soft tissue opacity structure in the cranioventral abdomen. This structure is easily mistaken for a mass or gastric foreign body. A left lateral film can resolve the dilemma. Both left and right lateral films are recommended in cases of suspected gastric foreign bodies.

CASE 10
SIGNALMENT: 2-year-old male domestic
    shorthair cat
REASON FOR PRESENTATION: chronic right
    forelimb lameness; hot, swollen, and painful
    carpus on physical examination

Figure 8.15 Dorsopalmar (A) and mediolateral (B) views of the carpus. There is focal, moderate to severe soft tissue swelling centered on the carpus. Irregular, poorly defined, and poorly mineralized new bone is present on the cranial aspect of the distal radius. Motheaten lysis of the distal radial epiphysis is visible. The small carpal bones are completely destroyed, and the joint has collapsed.

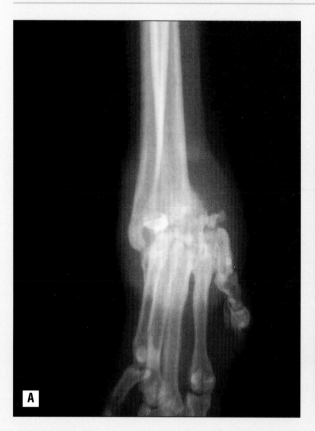
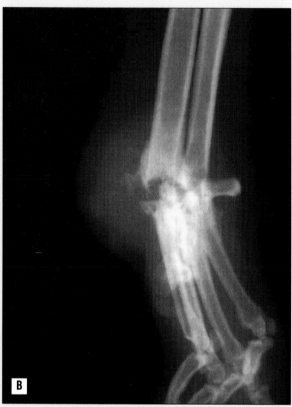

Diagnosis: aggressive erosive joint disease consistent with septic arthritis

Case comments: This is a very aggressive, destructive process. Only one joint is affected, so septic arthritis is the most likely diagnosis, in this case probably as a result of direct inoculation from a cat bite. Erosive disease affecting multiple joints may be the result of rheumatoid arthritis in dogs or periosteal proliferative polyarthritis in cats.

CASE 11

SIGNALMENT: 5-year-old domestic shorthair cat
REASON FOR PRESENTATION: history of chronic
vomiting, inappetence, and weight loss

Figure 8.16 On the right lateral radiograph (A), the stomach is enlarged and filled with uniform soft tissue opacity (arrows). On the left lateral radiograph (B), gas fills the lumen of the pylorus (★). The shape of the gas shadow is unusual, and there is apparent wall thickening. This appearance may be due to food adhered to the wall, however, and the interpretation must be made with care. The ventrodorsal radiograph (C) is unremarkable.

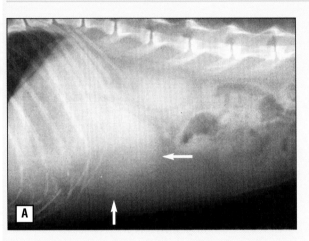

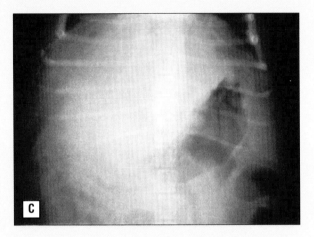

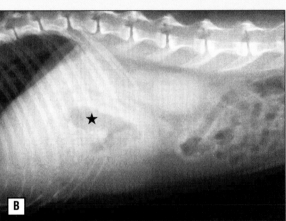

Figure 8.17 An ultrasound examination revealed diffuse moderate to severe thickening of the wall of the distal body and pyloric antrum of the stomach. The wall is diffusely hypoechoic with complete obliteration of wall layers. Note the bright hyperechoic stripe in this image, which represents the lumen. Thickened stomach wall is visible on both sides of the lumen.

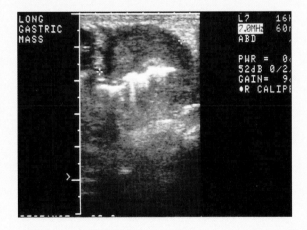

Diagnosis: infiltrative gastric mass, most likely neoplastic

Case comments: Lymphoma was diagnosed by fine-needle aspirate. This is the most common gastric tumor in cats. Adenocarcinomas are the most common gastric tumors in dogs.

CASE 12

SIGNALMENT: 11-year-old cocker spaniel dog
REASON FOR PRESENTATION: history of weight
loss and vomiting; cranial abdominal mass
palpated

Figure 8.18 Ventrodorsal (A) and lateral (B) views of the abdomen. An ovoid homogeneous soft tissue mass is seen in the craniodorsal abdomen on the lateral film. This displaces the intestine ventrally and caudally. A normal left kidney is present. In the ventrodorsal view, there is medial displacement of the ascending colon and descending duodenum in the right cranial abdominal quadrant. There is medial and caudal displacement of the small intestine.

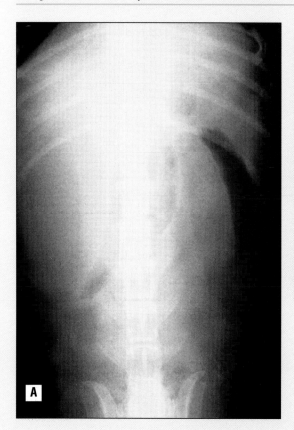

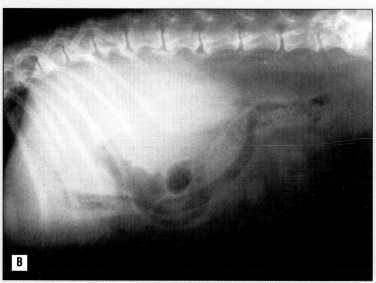

Diagnosis: right craniodorsal abdominal mass

Case comments: The right kidney is the most likely organ of origin. Other possible origins include the right adrenal gland and the caudate lobe of the liver. Either of these would probably have displaced the right kidney cau-

dally; thus, the absence of a visible right kidney makes it the most likely source of the mass. A large renal mass was confirmed on ultrasound and was found to be a carcinoma.

SIGNALMENT: 10-month-old bull terrier dog
REASON FOR PRESENTATION: right hind
lameness of 2 months' duration; mild tarsocrural
joint swelling noted

Figure 8.19 Dorsoplantar views of left (A) and right (B) tarsal joints. The left tarsus is normal. Note the normal contour of the medial trochlear ridge of the talus. A small bone fragment and corresponding defect are present at the proximal aspect of the medial trochlear ridge of the talus.

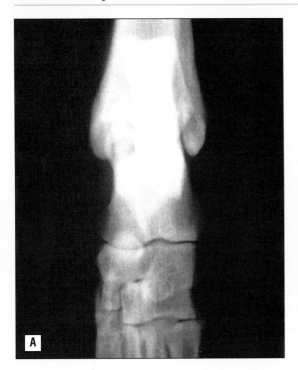

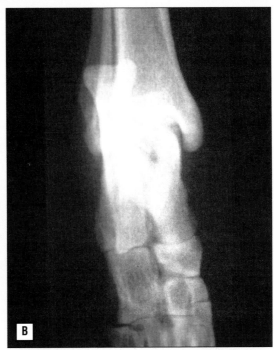

Figure 8.20 Sagittal plane reconstructed computed tomography image of the medial ridge of the talus. The computed tomography scan was performed to assess the size of the lesion and practicality of an arthroscopic procedure. This image shows a defect in the subchondral bone of the proximal aspect of the talus. A fragment of bone can be seen within the defect.

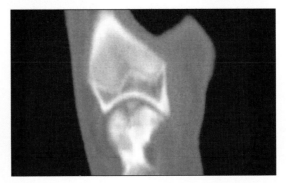

Diagnosis: osteochondritis dissecans of the medial trochlear ridge of the talus of the right tarsus

Case comments: The computed tomography image shows the size and precise location of the lesion more clearly than the radiographs.

CASE 14

SIGNALMENT: 12-year-old West Highland white terrier dog

REASON FOR PRESENTATION: history of vomiting and weight loss; palpable abdominal mass

Figure 8.21 Lateral (A) and ventrodorsal (B) abdominal radiographs of the dog. There is a homogeneous soft tissue mass in the cranioventral abdomen. The mass displaces the intestine dorsally and caudally. It lies at midline on the ventrodorsal film and causes caudal and rightward displacement of the intestine. Initial radiographic diagnosis: cranioventral abdominal mass. The spleen is the most likely organ of origin. Other possibilities include the liver, mesentery, or lymph node.

Figure 8.22 A and B, Ultrasonographic images of the mass shown in *Figure 8.21*. The mass had a mixed echoic parenchyma with multiple small cavitary areas. It originated from the tail of the spleen (arrows). The other abdominal organs were unremarkable. Ultrasonographic diagnosis: splenic mass.

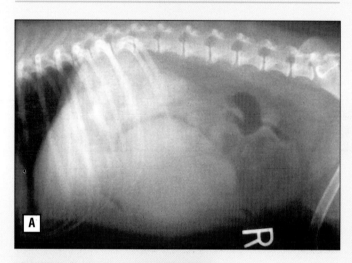

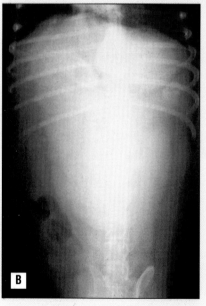

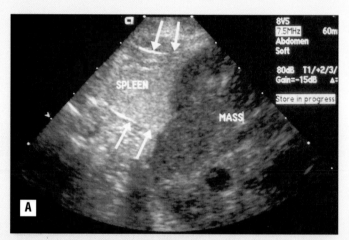

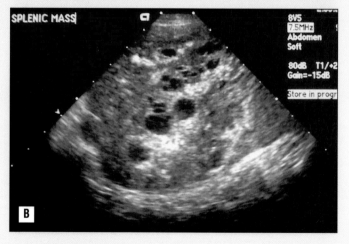

Diagnosis: splenic mass

Case comments: The appearance of the mass is quite nonspecific. On ultrasound images, splenic hemangiosarcomas and splenic hematomas show identical appearances similar to that of this mass. The dog's spleen was removed, and the histologic diagnosis was malignant histiocytosis.

radius and ulna. At the margins of the fractures, the new bone is irregularly margined and less well mineralized. These changes appear mildly aggressive, active, and chronic. New bone formation due to instability is usually confined to the area adjacent to the fracture. The extensive new bone formation that extends some distance from the fracture in this case indicates osteomyelitis.

Fig. 2.13....Mediolateral view of a normal stifle. The double-headed arrow indicates the location of the infrapatellar fat pad between the patellar ligament and the soft tissues of the stifle joint. The other arrow indicates the fat in the fascia at the caudal aspect of the stifle joint.

Fig. 2.14....Close-up ventrodorsal view of the left hip of a 7-year-old German shepherd dog. The acetabulum is shallow, and large osteophytes are present at the cranial and caudal acetabular rims and on the femoral neck. Note that the joint space is irregular. The cranial aspect of the joint space is markedly narrowed. This indicates destruction of the articular cartilage. Diagnosis: hip dysplasia, with moderate to severe degenerative joint disease.

Fig. 2.15....Craniocaudal view of the femur of a 4-year-old mixed-breed dog. A car had hit the dog approximately 4 months before presentation. There is a mid-diaphyseal fracture of the femur. Both the fracture ends are rounded with smoothly marginated, well-defined, well-mineralized, new bone formation. There is overriding of the fracture with proximal and lateral displacement of the distal fracture fragment. Diagnosis: hypertrophic nonunion.

Fig. 2.16....Mediolateral (A) and craniocaudal (B) views of the antebrachium of a 2-year-old Chihuahua dog. This dog had suffered radial and ulnar fractures 6 months before presentation. There is a healed malunion fracture of the distal radius with cranial angulation. The diaphysis of the ulna tapers to a point (arrow), and a large fracture gap is present. There is generalized loss of opacity in the small carpal bones and proximal metacarpals. Diagnosis: healed malunion radial fracture, atrophic nonunion ulnar fracture, and loss of bone opacity in the carpal bones due to disuse.

Fig. 2.17....Lateral view of the skull of an 11-year-old mixed-breed dog. There is diffuse loss of bone mineral. Note how the teeth appear quite opaque, and the bones are almost soft tissue opacity. Diagnosis: renal secondary hyperparathyroidism.

Fig. 2.18....Lateral view of the thoracolumbar spine of a 5-month-old domestic shorthair cat. There is poor mineralization of all the skeletal structures. The endplates of the vertebral bodies appear very opaque in comparison with the remainder of the spine, and there is poor contrast between the soft tissues and bones. These changes indicate greater than 70% loss of bone mineral content. Diagnosis: nutritional secondary hyperparathyroidism. (The owner had been feeding a diet consisting almost entirely of raw meat.)

Fig. 2.19....Mediolateral view of the antebrachium of an 11-year-old Irish setter dog. There is moderate soft tissue swelling of the antebrachium. Palisade-type new bone is notable along the metaphyses and diaphysis of the radius and ulna. This new bone is well mineralized and irregularly marginated. Notice how the epiphyses have been spared. Diagnosis: hypertrophic osteopathy. Thoracic radiographs revealed a pulmonary mass that was determined to be an adenocarcinoma.

Chapter 3: The Appendicular Skeleton

Fig. 3.1......Mediolateral view of the shoulder of a 6-month-old Labrador retriever dog. The caudal aspect of the humeral head is flattened and irregularly marginated. A thin, mineralized structure (arrows) is seen adjacent to the caudal humeral head. This represents a mineralized cartilaginous flap within the joint pouch. Diagnosis: shoulder OCD.

Fig. 3.2......Mediolateral (A) and caudocranial (B) views of the stifle of a 6-month-old Labrador retriever dog. The joint capsule bulges cranially, compressing the infrapatellar fat pad, and caudally, displacing the fat in the fascia (arrows), indicating there is moderate to severe joint effusion and/or capsular thickening. In the caudocranial view, the distal aspect of the lateral femoral condyle is flattened. Compare the appearance of the flat articular surface of the lateral femoral condyle to the rounded normal convex outline of the medial femoral condyle. A thin, mineralized structure is notable adjacent to the caudal aspect of the femoral condyles on the mediolateral view and represents a poorly mineralized flap of cartilage. Diagnosis: OCD of the lateral femoral condyle.

Fig. 3.3......Mediolateral view of the elbow of a Great Dane dog. A radiolucent line separates the anconeal process from the body of the ulna. Diagnosis: ununited anconeal process.

Fig. 3.4......Craniocaudal view of the elbow of a 7-month-old Labrador retriever dog. A small, shallow, concave defect can be seen in the articular surface of the medial aspect of the humeral condyle (arrow). A small, mineralized fragment is notable within this concave defect. Diagnosis: OCD of the distal humeral condyle.

Fig. 3.5......Flexed lateral (A) and craniocaudal (B) views of the elbow of a 10-month-old rottweiler dog. The long arrows indicate osteophyte formation on the anconeal process. The short arrows indicate sclerosis in the area of the anconeal process, which also represents osteophyte production. In the craniocaudal view, a moderately sized, pointed osteophyte is present on the medial coronoid process of the proximal ulna. There is no evidence of a UAP or an OCD lesion. As in most cases of fragmentation of the medial coronoid process, a distinct fragmented coronoid process cannot be identified. By eliminating UAP and OCD, FCP is the diagnosis by exclusion for a juvenile, large breed dog with DJD of the elbow. Diagnosis: elbow DJD presumed due to FCP. This diagnosis was confirmed by arthrotomy.

Fig. 3.6......Ventrodorsal view of the pelvis of a 2-year-old collie dog. Shown are normal coxofemoral joints. Note how the femoral heads are seated in the acetabula. The dorsal rim of the acetabula can be seen through the femoral heads and is lateral to the center point of the femoral heads. Dorsal acetabular coverage is approximately 60%. The joint space is uniform in width, and no periarticular osteophytes are visible.

Fig. 3.7......Ventrodorsal view of the pelvis of a 6-month-old mixed-breed dog. Both femoral heads are luxated; but, as yet, there is no evidence of DJD. Diagnosis: hip dysplasia.

Fig. 3.8......Ventrodorsal view of the pelvis of a 7-year-old mixed-breed dog. The film is slightly oblique, which can be determined by comparing the sizes of the obturator foramina. The larger foramen (in this case the left foramen) is rotated upward, away from the table. This rotation causes the acetabulum to appear deeper than it really is while making the contralateral acetabulum appear shallower. The right coxofemoral joint is moderately shallow. Large osteophytes can be noted at the cranial acetabular rim (arrow) and on the femoral neck between the greater trochanter and the femoral head (long arrow). Similar osteophyte formation is noted on the neck of the left femur. The joint space is uneven in both hip joints. Diagnosis: hip dysplasia and moderate DJD.

Fig. 3.9......Mediolateral view of the elbow of a 10-month-old mixed-breed dog. There is increased opacity within the proximal ulna. Compare the appearance of the medullary cavity of the ulna, where the endosteal surface of the cortex cannot be seen, to that of the radius. Diagnosis: panosteitis.

Fig. 3.10....Mediolateral view of the antebrachium of a 12-month-old Doberman pinscher dog. There is mottled increased opacity within the medullary cavity of the mid-diaphysis of the radius. Diagnosis: panosteitis.

Fig. 3.11....Mediolateral view of the distal humerus of a 15-month-old German shepherd dog. There is well-defined increased opacity within the medullary cavity of the distal third of the humeral diaphysis. Diagnosis: panosteitis. This lesion is well developed and chronic.

Fig. 3.12....Craniocaudal (A) and mediolateral (B) views of the distal antebrachium of a 5-month-old Weimaraner dog. Mild soft tissue swelling can be seen. There are poorly defined zones of lysis parallel to the physis within the metaphyses of the distal radius and distal ulna (long arrows). In the craniocaudal view, a linear focal mineralization is seen in the soft tissues at the lateral aspect of the distal ulnar metaphysis (short arrows). Less well-developed mineralization is seen at the caudal aspect of the ulna in the mediolateral view (short arrows). Diagnosis: hypertrophic osteodystrophy.

Fig. 3.13....Ventrodorsal view of the pelvis of a 12-month-old Yorkshire terrier dog. There is mild subluxation of the right femoral head, which is misshapen and has an uneven opacity. Diagnosis: idiopathic aseptic necrosis of the femoral head.

Chapter 4: The Axial Skeleton

Fig. 4.1......Lateral (A) and dorsoventral (B) views of the skull of a 6-month-old Scottish terrier dog. A large exostosis is noted on the left tympanic bulla (arrows). This new bone is very well mineralized and well defined, with smooth margins indicating the lesion is chronic. Note the normal triangular dark air shadow of the frontal sinuses on the lateral view. Diagnosis: craniomandibular osteopathy.

Fig. 4.2......Magnetic resonance images of the brain. A, Transverse T1-weighted image of the brain of a 12-year-old mixed breed dog that had a meningioma in the caudal fossa causing obstructive hydrocephalus. Note that both lateral ventricles are moderately dilated and that the cerebrospinal fluid is dark gray. The bones of the calvarium are black, and the subcutaneous fat is quite bright. B, Dorsal-plane T2-weighted image of a 6-year-old Siberian husky. This dog was evaluated for seizures, but both CT and MRI scans were normal. Note that cerebrospinal fluid and the aqueous and vitreous humors of the eye are bright. Cerebrospinal fluid can be seen surrounding the brain, and there is an appreciable difference between the gray and white matter of the cerebrum.

Fig. 4.3......Lateral view of the skull (A); rostrocaudal view of the frontal sinuses (B); and close-up, dorsoventral, intraoral view of the nasal chamber (C) of a 12-year-old mixed-breed dog. Note the increased soft tissue opacity within the frontal sinus on the lateral view. On the rostrocaudal view, the soft tissue opacity is seen to be within the left frontal sinus and the right is normal. Note the normal, fine, linear bony structures of the turbinates in the right nasal chamber on the intraoral film. The intraoral film shows homogeneously increased soft tissue opacity within the caudal portion of the left nasal chamber and complete destruction of the turbinates. Radiographic diagnosis: soft tissue mass with turbinate destruction in the left caudal nasal chamber, most likely neoplasia. This lesion was a nasal adenocarcinoma.

Fig. 4.4......Ventrodorsal open-mouth view of the nasal chambers of a 4-year-old pointer dog. There is increased lucency within the left nasal chamber, which appears quite black. There is complete destruction of the turbinates within the rostral and caudal portions of the left nasal chamber. Mild loss of opacity is also noted within the rostral nasal chamber on the right. Diagnosis: destructive rhinitis. Nasal aspergillosis was confirmed by endoscopy and serology.

Fig. 4.5......Transverse CT (A) and MR (B) images of the caudal nasal chamber of a normal 6-year-old Siberian husky. Note that the bones are quite white on the CT image. The fine scroll-like structures of the turbinates are clearly visible. This image has been adjusted to evaluate soft tissues, and fat within the orbit can be distinguished from the extra-ocular muscles. In the MR image, similar turbinate detail can be seen. The superior soft tissue imaging characteristics of this modality are evident in the ability to see the lens capsules.

Fig. 4.6......Ventrodorsal open-mouth view of the nasal chamber of a 10-year-old collie-cross dog (A) and transverse (B) and dorsal plane (C) MR images at the level of the eyes of the same dog. The radiograph shows an indistinct increased soft tissue opacity in the caudal nasal chamber on the right side. There is mild loss of the normal turbinate structures in this part of the nose. The MRI scan shows an inhomogeneous mass (★), which has destroyed parts of the turbinates within the caudal portion of the nasal chamber. Note how the extent in size of the mass is significantly better defined by the MRI scan. Diagnosis: caudal nasal mass. The histologic diagnosis was carcinoma.

Fig. 4.7......Transverse CT (A and B) and MR (C) images at the level of the tympanic bullae of a normal 6-year-old Siberian husky. A bone imaging protocol has been applied in image A, and the external ear canal is clearly seen. The fine detail of the wall of the bulla is also well demonstrated, as is the adjacent petrous temporal bone. All of the soft tissues are a uniform gray, however. The B image has been adjusted to evaluate soft tissues, and the fine detail of the bones cannot be seen as clearly. There are dark streaks within the brain in the caudal fossa; these are called beam-hardening artifacts. They occur when dense bone is imaged and render CT less suitable for evaluating the caudal fossa. The MR image (C) was obtained in a slightly different plane. Clarity of the ear structures is comparable to that of the CT scans. Note the superior image quality of the brain.

Fig. 4.8......Rostrocaudal open-mouth view (A) and dorsoventral view (B) of the tympanic bullae of an 8-year-old cocker spaniel dog. There is asymmetry of the tympanic bullae on the rostrocaudal and dorsoventral films. In both views, there is increased opacity within the left tympanic bulla (long arrows), with loss of the normal air shadow. The wall of the bulla is moderately thickened. The wall of the right bulla is thin and normal and contains a normal air shadow (short arrows). Diagnosis: chronic otitis media and bulla osteitis of the left ear.

Fig. 4.9......Lateral (A) and ventrodorsal (B) views of the cranial cervical spine of a 5-month-old Yorkshire terrier dog. The space between the spinous process of the axis and the arch of the atlas is widened, and there is slight malalignment of the atlantoaxial articulation on the lateral view. On the ventrodorsal view, no dens can be seen at the cranial aspect of the axis. Diagnosis: atlantoaxial subluxation.

Fig. 4.10....A and B, Lateral view of the thoracolumbar spine and lateral myelogram of an 11-year-old dachshund dog. There is narrowing of the L1-2 disk space (long arrow), and the associated intervertebral foramen (short arrow) and articular facet joint space are also reduced in size in comparison to adjacent disks (A). Increased opacity is noted within the intervertebral foramen at L1-2. Note the mineralized disk nucleus at T13-L1, which is contained within the disk space. Disk mineralization is a common finding in chondrodystrophic dogs. Positive contrast agent was injected into the subarachnoid space to outline the spinal cord, a myelogram. The myelogram (B) shows marked attenuation of the contrast-filled subarachnoid space centered over the L1-2 disk, confirming the presence of spinal cord compression. Diagnosis: L1-2 intervertebral disk prolapse.

Fig. 4.11....Lateral view of the cranial cervical spine of a 9-year-old beagle dog. A well-defined, ovoid, mineralized structure (arrows) is noted within the vertebral canal dorsal to the C2-3 disk space. The C2-3 disk space is moderately narrowed in comparison with the C3-4 and C4-5 disk spaces. Compare the relationship of the atlas to the axis with *Figure 4.7A and B*. Diagnosis: C2-3 disk prolapse.

Fig. 4.12....Lateral (A) and ventrodorsal (B) views of the cranial lumbar spine of a 9-year-old Bernese mountain dog. There is a focal, lytic, poorly defined lesion within the second lumbar vertebra seen on the lateral film (short arrows). Also on the lateral film, note the thin line of the normal floor of the vertebral canal in L3 (long arrows), which is absent in the second lumbar vertebra. In addition, there is irregularly margined, poorly mineralized, new bone formation along the ventral aspect of the body of L2. In the ventrodorsal view, the arrows indicate the normal left-side transverse process (L2) and normal right side pedicle of L3. The right-side transverse process and right pedicle of L2 are absent. Diagnosis: aggressive, mixed, productive and destructive lesion of the L2 vertebra. The histologic diagnosis was malignant histiocytosis.

Fig. 4.13....A and B, Lateral view of the caudal cervical spine and myelogram of a 6-year-old Doberman pinscher dog. The body of C6 has an abnormal form, appearing slightly wedge shaped. The C5-6 and C6-7 disk spaces are narrowed, especially at their ventral aspect. The body of C6 is tilted dorsally, and there is mild to moderate malalignment of the spine at C5-6. The myelogram demonstrates dorsal displacement and attenuation of the ventral contrast-filled subarachnoid space, indicating a disk protrusion at C6-7. No compression is noted at C5-6, but ventroflexed and dorsiflexed films are required to exclude compression because the lesions are often dynamic. Diagnosis: cervical spondylomyelopathy.

Fig. 4.14....Lateral view of the lumbar spine of an 8-year-old German shepherd dog. There is lysis of the endplates of the vertebral bodies and collapse of the intervertebral disk spaces. Moderate to severe sclerosis surrounds the disk spaces. At the L2-3 disk space, there is ill-defined lysis of the caudal endplate of L2 with a concave appearance and mild sclerosis of the adjacent vertebral body. That appearance indicates a recent lesion. There is more severe sclerosis adjacent to the lytic lesions of the other vertebral endplates indicating these lesions are chronic. Diagnosis: diskospondylitis at multiple sites. *Aspergillus* spp was cultured from the dog's urine.

Chapter 5: The Thorax

Fig. 5.1 ......Lateral (A) and VD (B) views of a normal 2-year-old rottweiler and lateral (C) and VD (D) views of a normal 2-year-old English bulldog. Note the difference in thoracic conformation. The rottweiler has a "standard" chest conformation with a thoracic cavity that is slightly deeper than it is wide. Note the shape and size of the heart. The bulldog has a thorax that is wide, shallow, and foreshortened in the cranial-to-caudal dimension. Its heart appears relatively larger in the DV view because it lies transversely across the thorax. The cranial border of the heart is partly obscured on the lateral view, which is a frequent finding in brachycephalic breeds.

Fig. 5.2 ......Lateral (A) and VD (B) views of the thorax of a normal 2-year-old domestic shorthair cat. The heart is slightly smaller than that of a normal dog. Note its somewhat lemonlike outline and slightly cranial tilt. A moderate amount of pericardial fat surrounds the heart on both lateral and VD views. Also note the normal appearance of the caudal lobar vessels.

Fig. 5.3 ......Close-up view of the right thoracic wall of a 3-year-old pug dog. There are transverse fractures of all of the ribs in this view. The fracture ends are sharp, and no evidence of new bone formation is noted. The lung lobe edges are separated from the thoracic wall by a thin band of fluid opacity. Fissure lines are seen between the right middle and caudal lung lobes. These findings indicate the presence of a small volume of fluid within the pleural cavity. This is most likely hemorrhage. Diagnosis: recent rib fractures and pleural effusion.

Fig. 5.4 ......Lateral (A) and VD (B) views of the thorax of an 8-year-old Dalmatian dog. A homogeneous, well-defined, round, soft tissue mass is seen in the craniodorsal thorax on the lateral film. The VD radiograph shows this to be in the right cranial hemithorax. There is leftward deviation of the trachea on the VD film and slight ventral deviation of the trachea on the lateral view. There is destruction of the proximal half of the right second rib indicating this mass originated in the thoracic wall rather in the lungs. Diagnosis: chest wall tumor. The histologic diagnosis was osteosarcoma.

Fig. 5.5 ......Lateral view of the trachea of a 9-year-old Yorkshire terrier dog. This is an inspiratory film. There is complete obliteration of the lumen of the caudal cervical trachea. Moderate narrowing of the intrathoracic trachea can also be noted. Diagnosis: extrathoracic tracheal collapse.

Fig. 5.6 ......Lateral thoracic views of a 7-year-old toy poodle dog. In the inspiratory view (A), the intrathoracic trachea and mainstem bronchi are normal in diameter. On expiration (B), there is almost complete obliteration of the mainstem bronchi and moderate narrowing of the intrathoracic trachea. Diagnosis: intrathoracic tracheal and mainstem bronchi collapse.

Fig. 5.7 ......Lateral view of the cranial thorax of a 4-year-old domestic shorthair cat. There is loss of normal air shadow of the trachea in the fourth intercostal space. The lumen is narrowed to approximately 20% of the original diameter at this site by focal soft tissue swelling originating from the ventral and dorsal tracheal walls (arrows). The narrowing appears to be circumferential. Diagnosis: focal tracheal stenosis. This lesion was the result of a previous traumatic tracheal laceration.

Fig. 5.8 ......Lateral view (A) with close-up (B) and VD view (C) with close-up (D) of the thorax of an 11-year-old bull terrier dog. There is a large soft tissue mass in the region of the tracheal bifurcation. This causes ventral displacement and compression of the mainstem bronchi indicated by the arrows in the lateral close-up image (B). In the VD image, the mass can be seen lying between the caudal lobar bronchi. In the VD view, there is lateral displacement of both the caudal mainstem bronchi (arrows, D), which are moderately to severely compressed . Diagnosis: severe enlargement of the tracheobronchial lymph nodes. The histologic diagnosis was adenocarcinoma.

Fig. 5.9 ......Left lateral view of the cranial thorax of a 3-year-old mixed-breed dog. There is homogeneous increased opacity within the peripheral zone of the right cranial lung lobe and middle and peripheral zones of the right middle lung lobe. Linear branching gas shadows (arrows) are noted within the affected lung. These are air bronchograms. Note that the vessels of the affected lobes are completely obscured and cannot be seen. The cranial border of the heart blends with the lung and is completely obliterated. Both of these findings are examples of a silhouette sign. The air bronchograms and silhouette signs indicate that this is an alveolar pattern. Diagnosis: bronchopneumonia.

Fig. 5.10 ....Close-up lateral (A) and VD (B) views of the thorax of a 6-year-old Siamese cat. In the lateral view, multiple ringlike or doughnut-type markings are noted within the pulmonary parenchyma (arrows). There is also a diffuse moderate increase in lung opacity. Note that pulmonary vessels can still be seen, although the smaller vascular structures are obscured by the increased opacity. In the VD view, thin, parallel, linear soft tissue structures are evident (arrows) in the periphery of the lung field. These are often referred to as "railroad tracks" or "tramlines." These findings are consistent with a bronchial pattern. Diagnosis: feline asthma.

Fig. 5.11 ....Lateral view of the thorax of a 10-year-old rottweiler dog. There are multiple, well-defined soft tissue nodules that range from 5 to 20 mm in size distributed throughout the lung parenchyma in a nodular interstitial pattern. These were metastases from a prostatic carcinoma.

Fig. 5.12....VD view of the right caudal lung field of a 12-year-old mixed-breed dog. There are multiple small pulmonary nodules throughout the visible lung field. These are miliary nodules, which are so numerous that the overall effect is like that of a snowstorm. In such cases, individual nodules are often easier to see at the periphery of the lung where relatively fewer lesions are superimposed on each other. These were metastases from a splenic hemangiosarcoma.

Fig. 5.13....Close-up view of the caudodorsal thorax. There is a diffuse increase in soft tissue opacity. This reduces the visibility of the normal pulmonary vasculature but does not completely obscure the larger vessels. The pattern is not characterized by nodules, doughnuts, or railroad tracks and is therefore considered an unstructured interstitial pattern. The diagnosis was pulmonary infiltrate with eosinophilia due to heartworm infestation.

Fig. 5.14....VD view of the thorax of a 4-year-old mixed-breed dog presented after an automobile accident. There is homogeneous increased soft tissue opacity within the caudal subsegment of the left cranial lung lobe. This results in obliteration of part of the outline of the left side of the heart indicating that the pattern is alveolar. Diagnosis: traumatic contusion.

Fig. 5.15....Right (A) and left (B) lateral views and a VD view (C) of the thorax of a springer spaniel dog. This homogeneous soft tissue opacity within the right cranial and middle lung lobes obliterates the right border of the heart. In the left lateral view, air bronchograms are visible within the middle and peripheral portions of the lung lobes indicating the presence of an alveolar pattern. Note that no abnormalities are evident on the right lateral film, as quite substantial abnormalities may be invisible if in the downside lung when taking lateral views. Both left and right lateral views should be obtained in cases of suspected pneumonia. There is a mediastinal shift with the heart displaced toward the right body wall. Diagnosis: bronchopneumonia.

Fig. 5.16....VD (A) and lateral (B) views of the thorax of a dog presented after multiple seizures. There is homogeneous increased soft tissue opacity in the middle and peripheral zones of the right caudal lung lobe. An air bronchogram is seen within this affected portion of lung in the VD view. In the lateral view, this portion of lung obliterates the outline of the crus of the diaphragm indicating an alveolar pattern. Based on the type of pattern and the location, noncardiogenic edema is considered most likely. Diagnosis: noncardiogenic edema due to status epilepticus.

Fig. 5.17....Lateral films of the thorax of a 3-year-old Doberman pinscher dog obtained at presentation (A) and at 12 (B) and 24 (C) hours after treatment. The trachea is displaced dorsally and runs parallel to the thoracic spine. The caudal border of the heart cannot be seen on the lateral view due to increased soft tissue opacity. Increased lung opacity also causes obliteration of the outline of the cupola of the diaphragm. Pulmonary vessels cannot be seen in the hilar region of the affected lung. This is an alveolar pattern. The cranial lung lobes and the periphery of the caudal lobes appear normal. On the second film, obtained 12 hours after diuretic therapy had commenced, the pulmonary opacity has decreased and the heart and diaphragm can be seen. A moderate, hazy, unstructured interstitial pattern persists. On the film obtained 24 hours after treatment, there has been complete resolution of the pulmonary pattern. Diagnosis: alveolar pattern with perihilar distribution and severe cardiomegaly consistent with cardiogenic pulmonary edema due to dilated cardiomyopathy. The edema resolved quickly in response to treatment.

Fig. 5.18....VD view of a 3-year-old mixed-breed dog that had been hit by a car a few hours previously. Gas can be seen outlining the lateral border of all the lung lobes in both the left and the right hemithoraxes. There is homogeneous increased soft tissue opacity within the lung lobes, and the left border of the heart blends with the affected lung. The increased pulmonary opacity is too great to be accounted for by the relatively small reduction in lung volume caused by the pneumothorax. This indicates the presence of a second process, which in this case is most likely a contusion due to trauma. Diagnosis: pneumothorax, partial lung atelectasis, and contusion.

Fig. 5.19....Lateral view of the thorax of an 11-year-old cocker spaniel dog. There is homogeneous increased soft tissue opacity in the cranioventral lung field. Multiple air bronchograms are seen within these lung lobes. The cranial border of the heart is partly obscured. This is an alveolar pattern. The location of the lesion is typical of bronchopneumonia or aspiration pneumonia. Neither disease correlated with the clinical presentation, however; and the dog did not respond to treatment. Histologic diagnosis: pulmonary lymphoma.

Fig. 5.20....Lateral (A), VD (B), and DV (C) views of the thorax of a 9-year-old golden retriever dog. In the lateral view, there is dorsal retraction of the ventral border of the lung. The outline of the heart and cupola of the diaphragm cannot be seen. In the VD view, the heart can be seen outlined by the lungs. There is retraction of the lungs from the thoracic wall, and fluid opacity can be seen in the fissures between the lung lobes and separating the lungs from the thoracic wall. On the DV film, the heart and cupola of the diaphragm are completely obscured. There is a fissure line between the right caudal and middle lung lobes. Diagnosis: moderate-volume pleural effusion.

Fig. 5.21....Lateral (A), DV (B), and horizontal-beam VD (C) views of the thorax of a 2-year-old mixed-breed dog. The heart is separated from the sternum and displaced dorsally by a large gas bubble. On the lateral film, the dorsal border of both the caudal lung lobes is outlined by air. Pulmonary markings are not seen in the caudodorsal periphery or ventral periphery of the thoracic cavity. This finding indicates there is a pneumothorax. On the DV film, gas can be seen outlining the left caudal lung lobe. The heart is shifted toward the right thoracic wall. Air bronchograms are seen within the left caudal lung lobe, which is of homogeneous soft tissue opacity, and within the right middle lung lobe and right cranial lung lobe, which obliterate the right border of the heart. These abnormalities indicate the presence of an alveolar pattern. On the horizontal-beam VD view of the thorax, the pleural cavity is filled with gas and devoid of any pulmonary markings. Diagnosis: traumatic pneumothorax with pulmonary contusions.

Fig. 5.22....Lateral view of the cranial thorax of a greyhound dog. Note that both the inner and outer margins of the dorsal and ventral tracheal walls are clearly visible. A number of large, tubular, soft tissue opacity structures are also visible in the cranial thorax ventral to the trachea. These are some of the large vessels located in the cranial mediastinum and are normally invisible radiographically. Diagnosis: pneumomediastinum.

Fig. 5.23....VD view of the thorax of a cat. There is homogeneous soft tissue opacification of the right hemithorax, and no normal lung is present. Possible causes for this include a mass or unilateral pleural effusion due to or accompanied by an inflammatory process. The heart is displaced leftward and touches the left thoracic wall, a mediastinal shift. The left lung appears normal. Diagnosis: unilateral pleural effusion. This was found to be a pyothorax by thoracocentesis.

Fig. 5.24....Lateral thorax. There is uniform moderate gaseous dilation of the thoracic esophagus. Note the combined tracheal and esophageal wall, which forms a soft tissue stripe. This should not be confused with gas within the mediastinum, which outlines the walls of the trachea. The caudal thoracic esophagus is seen as two, thin, soft tissue lines converging on the esophageal hiatus of the diaphragm. Diagnosis: generalized megaesophagus.

Fig. 5.25....VD view of the thorax of a 4-year-old boxer dog. There is severe generalized enlargement of the heart. Note that the cardiac apex has shifted to the right side of the thorax. This creates the impression of predominantly right-sided cardiomegaly, but the apical shift indicates left- sided enlargement.

Fig. 5.26....Lateral (A) and VD (B) views of the thorax of a German shepherd dog presented for weakness, vomiting, and polydipsia. In the lateral view, the heart measures two intercostal spaces wide, is lifted from the sternum by a pad of mediastinal fat, and is shorter than normal. In the VD view, the heart is small, measuring less than one third the width of the thorax. The pulmonary vessels are small and difficult to see. The lung fields are dark and uniformly hyperlucent. Diagnosis: microcardia and pulmonary underperfusion. The dog was found to have Addison's disease.

Fig. 5.27....Lateral (A) and VD (B) views of the thorax of a normal dog. The arrows and numerals indicate the clockface analogy used to describe the location of cardiac structures on both the VD and lateral films. The loca-

tions of the cardiac chambers and great vessels within the cardiac silhouette are indicated. AO = aorta, LA = left atrium, LV = left ventricle, RV = right ventricle, RA = right atrium, MPA = main pulmonary artery, LAA = left atrial appendage.

Fig. 5.28....Lateral (A) and VD (B) views of the thorax of a 14-year-old toy poodle. There is severe dorsal displacement of the trachea. The heart is widened, measuring four and one-half intercostal spaces on the lateral film and over two thirds the width of the thorax in the VD view. These changes indicate severe, generalized enlargement of the heart A triangular bulge is noted at the caudodorsal aspect of the heart on the lateral film, representing a severely enlarged left atrium. This bulge causes extreme dorsal displacement of the mainstem bronchi. The enlarged left atrium is seen as increased soft tissue opacity between the two mainstem bronchi at the caudal aspect of the heart on the VD view. The lungs are normal, and there is no evidence of cardiogenic edema. Diagnosis: generalized severe cardiomegaly with severe left atrial enlargement. Mitral valve endocardiosis and incompetence was confirmed on echocardiography.

Fig. 5.29....Lateral (A) and VD (B) views of the thorax of a 1-year-old mixed-breed dog. The right cardiac border is rounded and expanded on the VD view, and the heart has a reversed-D type appearance. On the lateral film, the cranial cardiac border is rounded and the heart is wider than normal, measuring almost four intercostal spaces. The cardiac apex is elevated from the sternum in the lateral view. Diagnosis: moderate right-sided cardiomegaly. Echocardiography revealed tricuspid valve dysplasia.

Fig. 5.30....Lateral (A) and VD (B) films of the thorax of a golden retriever dog. On the lateral film, the heart is widened, measuring almost four intercostal spaces. There is a bulge at the cranial aspect of the heart ventral to the trachea. In the VD view, the heart is elongated with a bulge of the cranial aspect at approximately the 12 o'clock position. The heart is also widened with a rounded left border. The lungs are normal. Diagnosis: enlargement of the aortic arch and mild cardiomegaly. Echocardiography confirmed an aortic stenosis.

Fig. 5.31....Lateral (A) and VD (B) films of the thorax of 1-year-old Pomeranian dog. On the lateral film, there is rounding and expansion of the cranial cardiac border. The heart measures four intercostal spaces wide. There is mild dorsal elevation of the trachea, and the caudal vena cava is distended. On the VD film, the heart is widened, measuring almost 80% the width of the thorax. The apex is displaced toward the left thoracic wall. The right cardiac border is rounded and almost touches the right thoracic wall. This gives the heart a reversed-D type appearance. There is a bulge at the 1 o'clock position in the area of the main pulmonary artery. Diagnosis: severe right-sided cardiomegaly with main pulmonary artery bulge. A pulmonic stenosis was confirmed by echocardiography.

Fig. 5.32....Lateral thorax of a normal dog. The cranial lobar arteries and veins are labeled.

Fig. 5.33....Lateral (A) and VD (B) views of the thorax of a 3-month-old springer spaniel dog. On the lateral view, there is severe, generalized enlargement of the heart. This is evidenced by dorsal displacement of the trachea and widening of the heart, which measured over six intercostal spaces. Increased pulmonary soft tissue opacity partly obscures the caudal cardiac border. In the VD view, the heart is partly obscured by increased pulmonary opacity. A bulge is noted in the 12 to 1 o'clock position on the cardiac outline (arrow). The lateral border of this bulge blends with the descending thoracic aorta. Air bronchograms are noted within the hilar and middle zones of the right caudal lung lobe, and the right caudal border of the heart is obscured indicating the presence of an alveolar pattern. Diagnosis: severe cardiomegaly with aortic enlargement and left-sided heart failure with alveolar pulmonary edema. A patent ductus arteriosus was found on echocardiography.

Fig. 5.34....Lateral (A) and VD (B) films of the thorax of a 12-year-old Pomeranian dog. On the lateral view, the heart is moderately taller than normal. A large bulge is seen at the caudodorsal aspect of the heart representing a severely enlarged left atrium (short arrow). There is dorsal displacement of the trachea, which is almost parallel to the thoracic spine. The left caudal lobar bronchus is also displaced dorsally and compressed by the severely enlarged left atrium (long arrow). On the VD film, the heart is widened and the left cardiac border is rounded and expanded, almost touching the left thoracic wall. Increased soft tissue opacity is seen between the two caudal stem bronchi superimposed on the caudal aspect of the heart almost on midline, representing the enlarged left atrium (short arrows). The lungs are normal with no evidence of left-sided cardiac failure. Diagnosis: moderate cardiomegaly with severe left atrial enlargement. Mitral endocardiosis was found on echocardiography.

Fig. 5.35....Lateral (A) and VD (B) films of a 10-year-old cocker spaniel dog. On the lateral film, there is moderate to severe enlargement of the heart, which measures almost five intercostal spaces wide. The heart is tall and displaces the trachea dorsally. There is also dorsal displacement of the stem bronchi by a large bulge in the area of the left atrium. On the VD film, the heart is widened and rounded. There is indistinct increased opacity of the lungs in the area of the hilus on the lateral film. On the lateral film, there is also mismatch of the cranial lobar vessels with the pulmonary vein (arrows), measuring twice the size of the corresponding artery. Diagnosis: severe cardiomegaly with severe left atrial enlargement, pulmonary venous congestion, and unstructured interstitial pattern in the

hilar region of the lung lobes. This most likely represents pulmonary edema. Dilated cardiopathy was found on echocardiography.

Fig. 5.36....Lateral (A) and VD (B) views of the thorax of an adult domestic shorthair cat. The heart is tall, displacing the trachea dorsally on the lateral film. It is also widened, measuring over three intercostal spaces wide. On the VD film, the heart is moderately to severely widened and the cardiac apex is displaced to the right of midline. There is a bulge at the 3 o'clock position of the heart on the VD view, representing enlargement of the left atrial appendage. Patchy increased opacity is present within the lungs, and the hilar and peripheral zones of the caudal lung lobes. This opacity is characterized by an unstructured interstitial pattern that coalesces to form a patchy alveolar pattern. Diagnosis: left-sided cardiomegaly with pulmonary edema. Hypertrophic cardiomyopathy was found on echocardiography.

Fig. 5.37....Lateral (A) and VD (B) radiographs of the thorax of a 6-year-old domestic shorthair cat. There is moderate to severe enlargement of the right caudal lobar artery, which is seen on the VD radiograph. A moderate, unstructured increase in soft tissue opacity is noted throughout the lung fields. Both heart size and shape are considered to be within normal limits. The arterial abnormality is indicative of heartworm infestation. The unstructured interstitial pattern is consistent with pulmonary infiltrate with eosinophilia. Diagnosis: heartworm disease.

Fig. 5.38....Lateral thoracic radiograph of a 6-year-old German shepherd dog. The dog had been treated for heartworm disease with an adulticide. There is increased soft tissue opacity in the periphery of the caudal lung lobe. A mottled inhomogeneous opacity partly obliterates the outline of the diaphragm. The increased opacity has a wedge shape, with the base towards the diaphragm and the apex towards the hilus of the lung. Diagnosis: pulmonary thromboembolism.

Fig. 5.39....Lateral (A) and VD (B) radiographs of the thorax of a 7-year-old cocker spaniel dog. The heart is severely enlarged, measuring four and one-half intercostal spaces wide and rounded on the lateral view. Also, the heart is tall causing severe dorsal displacement of the trachea. Similar severe enlargement of the heart silhouette is present in the VD view, with the heart contacting the right thoracic wall and almost contacting the left thoracic wall. No specific cardiac chamber bulges or great vessel enlargements are noted. The lungs are normal. The VD radiograph does not support the increased opacity in the caudal lung lobes on the lateral film. It is most likely an artifact caused by poor inspiratory effort. Diagnosis: pericardial effusion. The presence of a moderate volume of pericardial fluid was confirmed by echocardiography. No evidence of a tumor was found.

Fig. 6.1......Lateral radiograph of the abdomen of a domestic short-hair cat that had been attacked by a dog. Several loops of small intestine are noted ventral to the abdominal wall. The musculature of the ventral abdominal wall can be traced from the caudal abdomen as a thin soft tissue stripe ventral to the bladder wall. Diagnosis: ventral rupture.

Fig. 6.2......Lateral radiograph of the abdomen of a cat. There is complete absence of fat within the peritoneal and retroperitoneal cavities. No subcutaneous fat can be noted. The abdomen has a "tucked-up" appearance. There is complete absence of serosal detail within the abdomen. In this case, there is no abdominal detail because of the complete absence of fat. The shape of the abdomen is the clue that indicates the peritoneal cavity is not filled with fluid. Diagnosis: cachexia. The cat had chronic renal failure.

Fig. 6.3......Lateral view of the cranial abdomen of a cat. Notice the large amount of fat within the falciform ligament ventral to the liver. A large amount of retroperitoneal fat is also present outlining the kidneys. Note the sharp detail of the serosal borders of the small intestine of the ventral midabdomen. Diagnosis: normal (well-fed) cat.

Fig. 6.4......Lateral radiograph of the abdomen of a cocker spaniel dog presented collapsed from a gunshot wound. There is increased soft tissue opacity within the dorsal abdomen, obliterating the outline of the kidneys. The gastrointestinal tract is displaced ventrally and compressed by the expanded retroperitoneal space. Serosal detail is still visible in the ventral abdomen indicating this process is confined to the retroperitoneal space. In the caudal thorax, the margins of the lungs are separated from the thoracic wall by soft tissue opacity. A metallic object is noted dorsal to the caudal thoracic spine. Diagnosis: retroperitoneal fluid or mass and pleural fluid. The right ureter had been lacerated by a bullet, causing urine leakage into the retroperitoneal space.

Fig. 6.5......Lateral view of the abdomen of a 10-year-old domestic shorthair cat. Note the normal detail within the retroperitoneal space where fat clearly outlines both the kidneys. There is increased soft tissue opacity within the peritoneal cavity, which partly, but not completely, obliterates the serosal margins of the intestines. Diagnosis: moderate volume of peritoneal fluid.

Fig. 6.6......Lateral view of the abdomen of a 3-year-old Siamese cat. The abdomen is moderately pendulous. There is no fat within the retroperitoneal or falciform areas. No serosal detail can be seen. There is homogeneous soft tissue opacity within the abdomen. In this cat there is no body fat to supply serosal detail; but the abdomen is distended rather than thin, indicating the presence of fluid. Compare this with *Figure 6.1*. Diagnosis: moderate volume of peritoneal fluid and cachexia. The final diagnosis was feline infectious peritonitis.

Fig. 6.7......Lateral view of the abdomen of a 6-year-old mixed-breed dog. Note that there is a gas bubble in the craniodorsal abdomen, which outlines the caudal surface of the diaphragm and the serosal surface of the fundus of the stomach. A thin curvilinear gas pocket can also be seen between the body of the stomach and the liver in the cranioventral abdomen. Diagnosis: moderate to large volume of free peritoneal gas.

Fig. 6.8......Close-up view of the cranioventral abdomen of a German shorthaired pointer, which presented collapsed. There is increased soft tissue opacity within the peritoneal cavity, with moderately to severely reduced serosal detail. Multiple, small gas bubbles are seen scattered in the ventral abdomen. These are not contained within the small or the large intestine. Diagnosis: free peritoneal gas and peritoneal fluid. A perforated duodenal ulcer was also found at surgery.

Fig. 6.9......VD, horizontal-beam view of the abdomen of 7-year-old German shepherd cross-breed dog. A large gas pocket is evident beneath the body wall. Note that this radiograph was taken with the dog in right lateral recumbency. The two short arrows indicate the wall of the stomach, the lumen of which contains a small gas bubble. The long arrow indicates the spleen. Horizontal-beam films should be taken with the patient in left recumbency to prevent confusion with the gas pocket in the stomach. Diagnosis: free peritoneal air. At surgery a ruptured liver abscess was found.

Fig. 6.10....Lateral view of the cranial abdomen of a 1-year-old miniature schnauzer dog. Gas is present within the fundus and body of the stomach. The gastric axis is tilted cranially. The caudoventral margin of the liver does not extend to the edge of the ribs. Diagnosis: microhepatia. A portosystemic shunt was ligated at surgery.

Fig. 6.11....Lateral (A) and VD (B) views of the abdomen of an 8-year-old mixed-breed dog. There is caudal and dorsal displacement of the stomach and caudal displacement of the small intestine. The liver extends beyond the ribs, and the caudoventral margin of the liver reaches almost to the level of the umbilicus. On the VD film, there is caudal and leftward displacement of the intestines from the right, cranial, abdominal quadrant. Diagnosis: generalized hepatomegaly. Lymphoma was diagnosed on aspiration biopsy.

Fig. 6.12....Close-up view of the mid-ventral abdomen of an 11-year-old mixed-breed dog. The spleen is seen lying along the ventral abdominal wall. It extends caudally almost to the bladder. There is slight rounding of the caudal margin of the spleen. Diagnosis: moderate, generalized splenomegaly. Fine-needle aspirates from the spleen were consistent with lymphoid hyperplasia.

Fig. 6.13....Right lateral (A), VD (B), left lateral (C), and DV (D) views of the cranial abdomen of a dog. Note that gas fills the fundus and body of the stomach on the right lateral projection. On the VD projection, the body and pyloric antrum of the stomach are filled with gas. On the left lateral projection, gas is noted within the pylorus and also distends the descending duodenum. On the DV film, the gas is predominantly located within the fundus. Diagnosis: normal stomach.

Fig. 6.14....VD view of the cranial abdomen and positive gastrogram of a normal cat. Note the shape of the stomach compared with that of a dog (*Figure 6.13*). Puppies' stomachs have a similar appearance to the stomach of this cat. Diagnosis: normal stomach.

Fig. 6.15....DV (A) and right lateral (B) views of the cranial abdomen of an 8-year-old Gordon setter dog. On the right lateral film, the stomach is moderately distended with gas. The fundus (diamond) is located in the ventral abdomen and is displaced caudally. The pylorus (star) is located in the left cranial abdomen rather than on the right. Diagnosis: gastric dilatation-volvulus.

Fig. 6.16....DV view of the abdomen of a hound cross-breed dog. Only this radiograph was obtained due to the dog's distressed and painful condition. There is massive gaseous dilation of the stomach. The pylorus (star) is in a normal location in the right cranial abdomen, and the fundus is on the left. Diagnosis: severe gastric dilatation without volvulus.

Fig. 6.17....Lateral view of the abdomen of a 2-year-old Labrador retriever dog. There are multiple, moderately dilated segments of small intestine, indicated by the long double-headed arrows. Several of the loops are filled with material that resembles poorly formed feces, and some are distended with gas. The presence of fecal-like material within dilated small intestine is consistent with a subacute to chronic, distal, small intestinal obstructive lesion. The short double-headed arrow indicates the position for measuring the height of L5. All of these small intestinal segments exceed 1.6 times the height of L5. Approximately one third to one half of the small intestine is dilated. Diagnosis: distal small intestinal obstruction.

Fig. 6.18....Lateral (A) and VD (B) views of the cranial abdomen of a domestic shorthair cat. Abundant retroperitoneal fat outlines both kidneys. The kidneys are normal in size and shape and have smooth margins and uniform soft tissue opacity. Diagnosis: normal kidneys.

Fig. 6.19....VD view of the cranial abdomen of a cat. The right kidney is small and slightly irregularly shaped. A small irregularly shaped mineral opaque structure is seen in the area of the renal pelvis. The left kidney is at the lower end of the normal range and slightly irregularly shaped. Diagnosis: chronic renal disease.

Fig. 6.20....Lateral view of the abdomen of a cat. The small and large intestine are displaced ventrally and caudally by two homogenous, well-defined ovoid soft tissue masses in the dorsal midabdomen (arrows). Normal kidney shadows cannot be seen. Diagnosis: severe, bilateral renomegaly. Renal lymphoma was diagnosed by fine-needle aspirate.

Fig. 6.21....Lateral abdomen of a terrier cross-breed dog. Multiple, irregularly shaped, mineral opaque uroliths can be seen within the lumen of the urinary bladder. Note that there are multiple uroliths also within the penile urethra caudal to the os penis (arrow). In cases of suspected urolithiasis in male dogs, a film centered on the penile urethra, with the animal's legs pulled forward, should always be obtained. Diagnosis: urocystolithiasis and urethral obstruction by uroliths.

Fig. 6.22....Lateral view of the caudal abdomen of a boxer dog. There is cranial displacement of the bladder by a mildly to moderately enlarged, rounded prostate. The prostate has homogenous soft tissue opacity and has smooth margins. Note the normal triangular fat opacity between the caudoventral aspect of the bladder, cranioventral aspect of the prostate, and abdominal wall (arrow). There is no evidence of enlargement of the sublumbar lymph nodes. Diagnosis: moderate prostatomegaly. The final diagnosis was benign prostatic hyperplasia.

Fig. 6.23....VD view of the abdomen. There are homogeneous soft tissue structures in the left and right caudal abdomen. These structures have displaced the small intestine cranially and toward midline. This is a characteristic pattern of displacement caused by uterine enlargement. Diagnosis: moderate uteromegaly. Pyometra was diagnosed by ultrasound.

Fig. 6.24....Lateral view of the midabdomen of a dog. A soft tissue structure present in the mid-ventral abdomen causes cranial and dorsal displacement of the small intestine. Within the soft tissue structures, multiple, fetal, mineral skeletal structures can be seen. Diagnosis: pregnancy.

Chapter 7: Abdominal Ultrasound

Fig. 7.1......Transverse view of the liver of a normal dog. Note the liver parenchyma has a granular, slightly coarse, uniform echotexture. Two large blood vessels cross the field of view. The deeper vessel with the hyperechoic wall is a portal vein. The more superficial vessel is a hepatic vein. Normal hepatic arteries and biliary ducts are not visible. Diagnosis: normal liver.

Fig. 7.2......Transverse view of the liver of a normal dog. The ovoid, dark structure on the left of the image is a normal gallbladder. Note that the gallbladder contents are anechoic. Diagnosis: normal liver.

Fig. 7.3......Sagittal scan of the liver of a terrier dog. An irregularly marginated, bilobate, hyperechoic mass is noted within the liver parenchyma. Diagnosis: hyperechoic liver mass. On additional images, several similar masses were noted. The histologic diagnosis after biopsy was nodular hyperplasia.

Fig. 7.4......Sagittal image of the liver of a 15-year-old domestic shorthair cat. There is uniform increased echogenicity within the liver. The arrows outline the capsule of the liver; and, superficial to that location, there is falciform fat. Normally the falciform fat is more echogenic than the liver. The portal veins cannot be seen due to the increased parenchymal echogenicity. Diagnosis: uniformly hyperechoic liver. The cytologic diagnosis was hepatic lipidosis.

Fig. 7.5......Dorsal plane image in the left cranial abdomen of a normal dog. The spleen is visible in the near field. A single splenic vein can be seen within the splenic parenchyma and penetrating the capsule of the spleen at the hilus. The bright hyperechoic line to the right and below the spleen is gas and fecal material within the colon. Diagnosis: normal spleen.

Fig. 7.6......Sagittal image of the tail of the spleen in a poodle dog. A solitary, well-defined, hypoechoic nodule is seen within the parenchyma of the spleen. Diagnosis: splenic nodule. The cytologic diagnosis was extramedullary hematopoiesis.

Fig. 7.7......Sagittal image of the spleen of a Persian cat. The splenic parenchyma is mottled with multiple, small, hypoechoic nodules. The remaining splenic parenchyma is identical in appearance. Diagnosis: multiple nodules. The cytologic diagnosis was lymphoma.

Fig. 7.8......Sagittal image of the left kidney of a normal dog. Note that the medulla is dark, almost anechoic. The cortex is uniformly echogenic with a fine granular echotexture. Diagnosis: normal kidney.

Fig. 7.9......Sagittal plane image of the left kidney of a cat. The medulla is almost anechoic, and there is sharp distinction between the medulla and cortex. The cortex is more echogenic than is normally seen in a dog. This is due to fat deposition within tubular cells, which is normal in cats. Diagnosis: normal kidney.

Fig. 7.10....Sagittal image of the kidney of a 3-year-old Persian cat. No normal renal architecture is seen. Multiple, thin-walled, cystic structures that contain anechoic or mildly echogenic fluid are notable. Diagnosis: polycystic kidney disease. The sonographic appearance of the right kidney was similar.

Fig. 7.11....Sagittal plane image of the left kidney of a 2-year-old German shepherd dog. There is an intense increase in echogenicity within the renal cortex. Also there is less dramatic increase in echogenicity within the medulla. The kidney is outlined by a moderate to large volume of anechoic fluid. Diagnosis: increased renal and medullary echogenicity. This was a case of ethylene glycol intoxication.

Fig. 7.12....Sagittal (A) and transverse (B) images of normal small intestine of a dog. Note the alternating hyper- and hypoechoic bands within the wall of the intestine, which is best seen on the sagittal image. In the transverse image, the intestine resembles a coffee bean. Diagnosis: normal intestine.

Fig. 7.13....Transverse plane image from the ventral midabdomen of a dog. Two moderately dilated, fluid-filled segments of small intestine are evident. In real-time imaging, there was no evidence of peristalsis. Several other simi-

lar loops were noted. There were also several loops of normal small intestine. Diagnosis: regional, moderate, small intestinal dilation. An intestinal obstruction was confirmed surgically.

Fig. 7.14....Sagittal image of the bladder of a 6-year-old bichon frisé. Three hyperechoic structures are seen in the dependent portion of the urinary bladder. Dark streaks are visible deep in these hyperechoic structures, representing acoustic shadowing. Diagnosis: urocystolithiasis.

Fig. 7.15....Sagittal image of the bladder of a 5-year-old Maine coon cat. There is moderate thickening of the urinary bladder wall, which measures 3 to 4 mm thick. A moderate amount of sediment is seen in the dependent portion of the urinary bladder. There is an indistinct outpouching from the bladder lumen at the apex of the bladder. Diagnosis: chronic severe cystitis with suspicion of a urinary bladder diverticulum, such as a urachal remnant. This was confirmed at surgery.

Fig. 7.16....Sagittal plane image of the neck of the bladder of a 10-year-old beagle dog. A mass of homogeneous echogenicity is indicated, outlined by long arrows. This appears to originate from the ventral wall of the neck of the bladder. The arrowhead indicates the vesicourethral junction. The mass has a homogeneous echogenicity with hyperechoic mucosal border. Diagnosis: bladder neck mass. A transitional cell carcinoma was diagnosed on aspiration biopsy.

Fig. 7.17....Transverse scan of the uterus of an 8-year-old greyhound dog. The uterus is moderately enlarged and the uterine horns are distended with mildly echoic to anechoic fluid. Diagnosis: pyometra.

Fig. 7.18....Ultrasound image of a canine fetus at approximately day 30 of gestation. This is a sagittal plane fetal image. The small, rectangular, hyperechoic structures represent the vertebrae. The heart can be seen surrounded by lungs. In real-time imaging, the heartbeat was detected. The liver can also be identified in this image. Diagnosis: normal pregnancy.

Fig. 7.19....Transverse image of the prostate of a recently neutered 2-year-old springer spaniel dog. The prostate is small, measuring approximately 1.5 cm in width, and has a slightly inhomogeneous hypoechoic echogenicity. The capsule is smooth and even. Diagnosis: normal prostate.

Fig. 7.20....Sagittal image of the prostate of a 7-year-old terrier cross-breed dog. The prostate is enlarged, measuring 3 cm in depth. The parenchyma has a mottled, hypoechoic appearance. Diagnosis: prostatomegaly with abnormal parenchyma. Prostatitis was diagnosed by aspiration biopsy.

Fig. 7.21....Sagittal image of the testicle of a 10-year-old German shepherd dog. A solitary, well-defined, hypoechoic nodule is present within the parenchyma of the caudal pole of the testicle. Note the hyperechoic structure at that center of the testicle, which is the mediastinum testis. Diagnosis: testicular tumor.

Fig. 7.22....Scan of the left dorsal midabdomen of an 8-year-old dachshund dog. The aorta (AO) is seen as a dark stripe that stretches obliquely across the image. The arrows indicate the left renal artery. Cranial to the artery and lateral to the wall of the aorta, the adrenal gland is seen as a well-defined, peanut-shaped, hypoechoic structure. The size of the adrenal gland is within normal limits. Diagnosis: normal left adrenal.

Fig. 7.23....Scan of the right cranial abdomen of a beagle dog. In the near field, the caudal vena cava is compressed by transducer pressure. The well-defined, hypoechoic, peanut-shaped structure dorsal to the caudal vena cava is the right adrenal gland. The size and echogenicity are within normal limits. Diagnosis: normal right adrenal gland. Note the close relationship to the caudal vena cava.

Fig. 7.24....Dorsal plane image of the right abdomen of a dachshund dog. A well-defined, mixed, echogenic mass is seen at the lateral aspect of the caudal vena cava (CVC). The mass was in the area of the right adrenal gland, and a normal right adrenal gland could not be identified. Diagnosis: right adrenal gland mass.

Fig. 7.25....Sagittal plane image of the right cranial quadrant of a 6-year-old mixed-breed dog. In the near field, there is a segment of descending duodenum. Between the two cursors deep to the duodenum, there is a portion of the right limb of the pancreas. The pancreaticoduodenal vein is seen as two, parallel, hyperechoic lines in the center of that portion of the pancreas. Diagnosis: normal pancreas.

Fig. 7.26....Sagittal plane image of the right cranial quadrant of a 5-year-old terrier cross-breed dog. The descending duodenum is in the near field. Deep to the descending duodenum, there is an irregularly marginated, hypoechoic structure. This is surrounded by intensely hyperechoic fat. The hypoechoic structure represents a moderately to severely enlarged pancreas. The hyperechoic tissue is reactive and inflamed fat. Diagnosis: moderate to severe pancreatitis.

Fig. 7.27....Sagittal plane image of the midabdomen of a cat. Multiple, well-defined, ovoid, hypoechoic structures are evident, surrounded by small intestine. These have uniform echogenicity. Diagnosis: moderately to severely enlarged mesenteric lymph nodes. Lymphoma was diagnosed by aspiration biopsy.

Chapter 8: Case Studies

Fig. 8.1......Craniocaudal view of the distal antebrachium and carpus of the dog. A mixed productive and destructive lesion is seen within the distal diaphysis and metaphysis of the radius. There is moth-eaten lysis of the radius. Irregularly marginated, well-mineralized new bone can be seen along the medial cortex of the distal radius. The location and appearance of this lesion are consistent with a primary malignant bone tumor. There is, however, also a destructive lesion within the proxi-

mal portion of the fifth metacarpal bone and complete lysis of the affected portion of the metacarpal. The presence of two lesions is atypical for a primary malignant bone tumor and suggests metastatic neoplasia or disseminated osteomyelitis. A bone scan was performed to evaluate the skeleton.

Fig. 8.2......Lateral skeletal scintigraphy images of the dog's right and left forelimbs and the thorax. There is intense focal tracer accumulation in the distal left antebrachium (1) and proximal left metacarpus (2). A focal area of increased uptake is also noted in the area of the olecranon of the left ulna (3). The focal radiotracer accumulation in the midportion of the right antebrachium (4) represents contamination from the intravenous injection of the radioactive tracer. A mild to moderate focal increased uptake can also be identified in the right eighth rib. Further, focal increased uptake is present in two sites in the cranial thoracic spine.

Fig. 8.3......Lateral view of the left elbow. A moth-eaten lytic lesion is noted within the olecranon. This has an ill-defined border and no evidence of new bone production. The appearance is similar to the fifth metacarpal lesion shown in *Figure 8.1.*

Fig. 8.4......Close-up view of the right side of the thorax. Smoothly marginated new bone formation is notable on the medial aspect of the right eighth rib. No evidence of bone lysis is visible.

Fig. 8.5......Craniocaudal (A) and lateral (B) views of the distal antebrachium of the dog. These radiographs were obtained immediately after surgical repair of oblique fractures of the radius and ulna. A bone plate and multiple screws have been used to stabilize the fracture. The alignment and reduction of the fracture are satisfactory.

Fig. 8.6......Lateral (A) and craniocaudal (B) views of the distal antebrachium of the dog. The second set of radiographs was obtained 6 weeks after the initial repair. There is moderate to severe soft tissue swelling surrounding the distal antebrachium. Abundant, irregularly marginated, poorly to moderately well-mineralized new bone is noted on the distal radius and ulna extending some distance from the fractures.

Fig. 8.7......Rostrocaudal view of the frontal sinus (A), ventrodorsal open-mouth view of the nasal chambers (B), and oblique view of the right frontal sinus (C). There is increased soft tissue opacity within the right frontal sinus and ill-defined loss of bone at the lateral aspect of the sinus. The oblique view demonstrates a large defect in the frontal bone, which has irregular moth-eaten margins. There is soft tissue swelling superficial to this defect. The ventrodorsal open-mouth view (B) demonstrates increased soft tissue opacity within the right caudal nasal chamber with destruction of the nasal and ethmoid turbinates.

Fig. 8.8......A magnetic resonance scan was performed for treatment planning. In this sagittal plane image, the tumor mass is indicated by the star. The arrows indicate extension of the tumor mass into the calvarium.

Fig. 8.9......Lateral (A) and ventrodorsal (B) views of the thorax. There is a homogeneous increased soft tissue opacity in the cranial thorax, which obliterates the outline of the heart. The trachea is displaced dorsally and to the right. On the ventrodorsal view, this soft tissue mass is seen to be on midline. It displaces the left and right cranial lung lobes caudally and laterally.

Fig. 8.10....Ventrodorsal (A) and lateral (B) radiographs of the dog's thorax. In the ventrodorsal view, there is increased soft tissue opacity in the left caudal hemithorax, which obliterates the outline of the heart and the left side of the diaphragm. On the lateral film, there is increased soft tissue opacity in the caudal thorax, which obliterates a portion of the outline of the cupola of the diaphragm and the caudal cardiac border. The two arrowheads indicate the diaphragmatic crura. A gas-filled structure is noted in the caudodorsal thorax (longer arrows). This represents the fundus of the stomach, which lies cranial to the diaphragmatic crura.

Fig. 8.11....Lateral (A) and ventrodorsal (B) films of the thorax. The cranial cardiac border is rounded and the heart is widened on the lateral radiograph. The right cardiac border is rounded on the ventrodorsal view, and the heart has a reversed-D type appearance. A large bulge is seen at the 1 o'clock position on the heart—the location of the main pulmonary artery—on the ventrodorsal view. There is moderate to severe enlargement of the left and right caudal lobar arteries (arrows). There is a moderate increase in unstructured pulmonary opacity. This is most severe at the periphery of the lung fields on the lateral film.

Fig. 8.12....Lateral (A) and ventrodorsal (B) views of the thorax. There is severe enlargement of the heart silhouette, which causes dorsal displacement of the trachea. On the ventrodorsal view, the heart contacts both thoracic walls. There are multiple tubular gas-filled structures at the caudoventral aspect of the heart silhouette on the lateral film. These are loops of small intestine, some of which are mildly to moderately dilated. In the ventrodorsal view, there is cranial displacement of the body of the stomach in the left cranial abdomen. The cupola of the diaphragm blends with the outline of the heart.

Fig. 8.13....Lateral (A) and dorsoventral (B) views of the thorax. In the lateral view, the diaphragm is pushed caudally and flattened. In the ventrodorsal view, the thorax is wide causing a barrel-chested appearance. There are multiple doughnut-type markings within the lung fields, which indicates the presence of a bronchial pattern. The lung fields are markedly overinflated.

Fig. 8.14....Left (A) and right (B) lateral radiographs of the cranial abdomen of the dog. The right lateral radiograph is normal. On the left lateral radiograph, a homogeneous soft tissue opacity structure is noted within the lumen of the stomach (arrows). Note the normal gas-filled pylorus in this view (★).

Fig. 8.15....Dorsopalmar (A) and mediolateral (B) views of the carpus. There is focal, moderate to severe soft tissue swelling centered on the carpus. Irregular, poorly defined, and poorly mineralized new bone is present on the cranial aspect of the distal radius. Moth-eaten lysis of the distal radial epiphysis is visible. The small carpal bones are completely destroyed, and the joint has collapsed.

Fig. 8.16....On the right lateral radiograph (A), the stomach is enlarged and filled with uniform soft tissue opacity (arrows). On the left lateral radiograph (B), gas fills the lumen of the pylorus (★). The shape of the gas shadow is unusual, and there is apparent wall thickening. This appearance may be due to food adhered to the wall, however, and the interpretation must be made with care. The ventrodorsal radiograph (C) is unremarkable.

Fig. 8.17....An ultrasound examination revealed diffuse moderate to severe thickening of the wall of the distal body and pyloric antrum of the stomach. The wall is diffusely hypoechoic with complete obliteration of wall layers. Note the bright hyperechoic stripe in this image, which represents the lumen. Thickened stomach wall is visible on both sides of the lumen.

Fig. 8.18....Lateral (A) and ventrodorsal (B) views of the abdomen. An ovoid homogeneous soft tissue mass is seen in the craniodorsal abdomen on the lateral film. This displaces the intestine ventrally and caudally. A normal left kidney is present. In the ventrodorsal view, there is medial displacement of the ascending colon and descending duodenum in the right cranial abdominal quadrant. There is medial and caudal displacement of the small intestine.

Fig. 8.19....Dorsoplantar views of left (A) and right (B) tarsal joints. The left tarsus is normal. Note the normal contour of the medial trochlear ridge of the talus. A small bone fragment and corresponding defect are present at the proximal aspect of the medial trochlear ridge of the talus.

Fig. 8.20....Sagittal plane reconstructed computed tomography image of the medial ridge of the talus. The computed tomography scan was performed to assess the size of the lesion and practicality of an arthroscopic procedure. This image shows a defect in the subchondral bone of the proximal aspect of the talus. A fragment of bone can be seen within the defect.

Fig. 8.21....Lateral (A) and ventrodorsal (B) abdominal radiographs of the dog. There is homogeneous soft tissue mass in the cranioventral abdomen. The mass displaces the intestine dorsally and caudally. It lies at midline on the ventrodorsal film and causes caudal and rightward displacement of the intestine. Initial radiographic diagnosis: cranioventral abdominal mass. The spleen is the most likely organ of origin. Other possibilities include the liver, mesentery, or lymph node.

Fig. 8.22....A and B, Ultrasonographic images of the mass shown in *Figure 8.21*. The mass had a mixed echoic parenchyma with multiple small cavitary areas. It originated from the tail of the spleen (arrows). The other abdominal organs were unremarkable. Ultrasonographic diagnosis: splenic mass.

-A-

air bronchogram: radiographic appearance of an air-filled bronchus surrounded by fluid-filled airspaces; visible as a branching dark gray line against uniform white lung tissue; considered the gold standard radiographic sign of the alveolar pattern but not always present.

alveolar pattern: cloudy to dense opacities that obscure vascular markings on thoracic radiographs; air that normally fills the alveoli is replaced by fluid or is displaced, in the case of atelectasis, due to collapse.

anechoic: in ultrasonography, free of echoes or without echoes; appears black. This is the only absolute term used to describe echogenicity.

attenuation: the process by which a beam of radiation is reduced in energy when passed through tissue or other material.

-B-

bronchial pattern: thickening of the bronchial walls seen as railroad tracks/tramlines (side-on bronchi) or doughnuts (end-on bronchi). Thickened walls of the major bronchi in the hilar zone are abnormal and are considered the most useful sign of bronchial disease. Bronchi in the mid and peripheral zones, which are normally invisible, are seen.

-D-

delayed union: slower than usual healing of a fractured bone.

-G-

gravel sign: an accumulation of small mineral fragments seen in the gastrointestinal tract proximal to a chronic partial obstruction due to sedimentation of heavier, indigestible food particles.

-H-

hyperechoic: in ultrasonography, a tissue or organ that produces echoes of higher amplitude or density in comparison with the normally expected appearance of a reference tissue or organ.

hyperlucent: a radiographic region showing greater than normal film blackening from increased passage of x-rays.

hypoechoic: in ultrasonography, a tissue or organ that produces echoes of lower amplitude or density in comparison to the normally expected appearance of a reference tissue or organ.

-I-

interstitial pattern: one of several pulmonary radiographic patterns associated with interstitial infiltration or thickening, including a nodular pattern and an unstructured pulmonary soft tissue pattern. The nodular pattern is characterized by multiple soft tissue nodules from 2 to 3 mm to 2 to 3 cm. An unstructured pattern is a poorly defined, hazy increase in opacity that causes the lung to appear too light, sometimes called the cotton candy effect.

isoechoic: in ultrasonography, a tissue or organ that produces echoes of equal amplitude or density in comparison to a reference tissue or organ.

-J-

joint mice: mineralized cartilaginous flap or osteochondral fragments.

-L-

long-scale contrast: numerous shades of gray in a black-and-white image, gradually changing from light to dark; obtained with a high kV(p) and low mA technique.

-M-

malunion: imperfect union of a fractured bone resulting in deformity or a crooked limb.

-N-

nonunion: failure of the ends of a fractured bone to unite.

-O-

opacity: radiographically, opacity is related to the ability to absorb x-rays. Increasing opacity results in greater x-ray absorption and a lighter appearance on the radiograph.

-R-

radiopharmaceutical uptake: absorption of a radioactive drug into tissue for temporary retention, to obtain images of internal organs or structures.

-S-

sclerosis: increased opacity of bone.

short-scale contrast: little gradation in shades of gray in a black-and-white image; obtained with low kV(p) and high mA technique.

signal intensity: a measure of the strength of the radio signal emitted by the body in magnetic resonance imaging. Tissues or organs with greater signal intensity appear brighter in the images.

silhouette sign: border obliteration that occurs radiographically when two objects of the same opacity are in contact, concealing the edges of both.

Burk RL, Ackerman N. *Small Animal Radiology and Ultrasonography: A Diagnostic Atlas and Text.* Philadelphia, Pa: WB Saunders Co; 1996.

Farrow CS, Green R, Shively M, eds. *Radiology of the Cat.* St Louis, Mo: Mosby; 1994.

Kealy JK, McAllister H. *Diagnostic Radiology and Ultrasonography of the Dog and Cat.* Philadelphia, Pa: WB Saunders Co; 2000.

Kealy JK, ed. Symposium on radiology. *Vet Clin North Am Small Anim Pract.* 1982;12.

Lavin LM. *Radiography in Veterinary Technology, 2nd Edition.* Philadelphia, Pa: WB Saunders Co; 1999.

Morgan JP. *Radiology of Veterinary Orthopedics.* Napa, Ca: Venture Press; 1999.

Morgan JP, Leighton RL. *Radiology of Small Animal Fracture Management.* Philadelphia, Pa: WB Saunders Co; 1995.

Morgan JP. *Techniques of Veterinary Radiography.* 5th ed. Ames, Ia: Iowa State University Press; 1993.

Nyland TG, Mattoon JS, eds. *Veterinary Diagnostic Ultrasound.* Philadelphia, Pa: WB Saunders Co; 2001.

Suter PF, ed. Symposium on radiology. *Vet Clin North Am Small Anim Pract.* 1974;4.

Thrall DE, ed. *Textbook of Veterinary Diagnostic Radiology.* Philadelphia, Pa: WB Saunders Co; 2002.

Subject Index

We've seen the future.
And it's just about to enter his stomach.

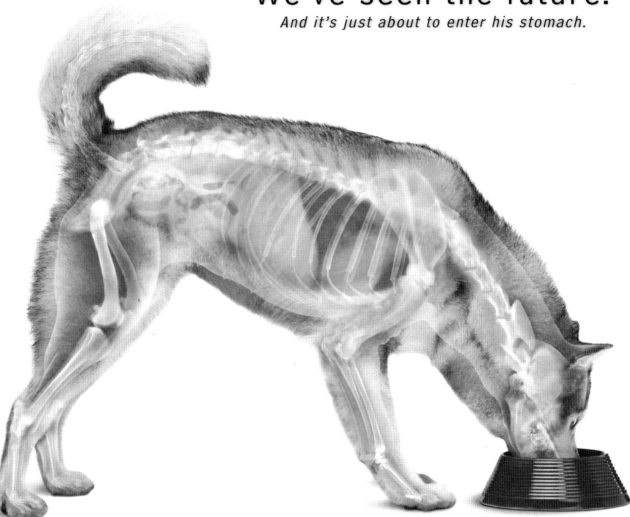

Bold new research is starting to reveal the full power of nutrition. At Purina, we were the first to use low-molecular-weight protein to control canine food allergies. The first to formulate a diet that works with a cat's metabolism to dramatically reduce insulin needs in some diabetic cats. The first to incorporate medium-chain triglycerides in canine diets to relieve gastrointestinal distress. And the first to use high protein levels to sustain lean body mass during weight loss. With breakthroughs like these, it's worthwhile taking a second look at the diets you put to work in your patients.